DATE		

For Mothers
&
Daughters

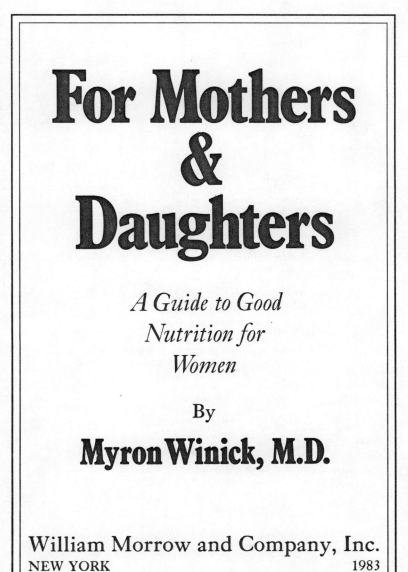

For Mothers & Daughters

*A Guide to Good
Nutrition for
Women*

By

Myron Winick, M.D.

William Morrow and Company, Inc.
NEW YORK   1983

Library of Congress Cataloging in Publication Data

Winick, Myron.
For mothers and daughters.

Includes index.
1. Women—Nutrition. I. Title.
TX361.W55W56 1983   613.2'088042   83–693
ISBN 0-688-01837-8

Printed in the United States of America

First Edition

1 2 3 4 5 6 7 8 9 10

BOOK DESIGN BY BLACKBIRCH GRAPHICS, BETHLEHEM, CONNECTICUT

This book is dedicated to
Ruth Winick, my mother,
and Elaine Winick, my wife,
the two most important women in my life.

———————

The author wishes to thank Ms. Elizabeth Frost Knappman for her suggestions and advice, and Mr. Ken Lane for organizing and editing the manuscript. Also, a special thanks to Ms. Maudene Nelson, who supplied the menus for the diets used in the book.

Contents

CHAPTER 1

How Women Are Different

More than one-third of the female population of the United States is deficient in one or more nutrients. By contrast, it is extremely rare for an adult male in our society to be deficient in any nutrient. And although women generally need fewer calories and therefore less food than men to fulfill their energy requirements, they need more of certain nutrients during their reproductive years.

On the far wider scale of life itself, a woman's nutrient requirements, because of the cyclic nature of her biology, will vary much more than those of a man. And since nutrients are supplied by food, and food is consumed for many reasons other than its nutritional content, some nutrients in a woman's diet are likely to be in constant short supply while others will probably be overabundant. In fact, women are the main target of food advertising both because of their own potential nutritional problems and because it is they who usually buy the family food. Moreover, certain elements in modern women's lifestyles make it easier for them to develop particular nutrient deficiencies.

All of these factors, working together, have led to an array of nutritional problems specific to women.

For example, while dietary excess is a common problem among both men and women in the Western world, the most important excess among women is in calories, followed by salt and fat, whereas among men, fat and salt take a close first and second place, with calories taking a more distant third. During a woman's reproductive years, the most obvious examples of lifestyle customs that can interfere with her biological needs are the use of the contraceptive pill to prevent pregnancy and the complete suppression. of lactation through pills that dry up the breast-milk supply, with the infant being bottle fed instead. The use of oral contraceptives can decrease the requirements for some nutrients and increase those for others, while a woman who does not breast feed will have to deal with the ten pounds of fat that accumulate during pregnancy specifically for the purpose of lactation.

Beyond this, the repeated loss and regaining of weight before or between pregnancies can deplete a woman nutritionally and affect her pregnancy outcome, her ability to produce breast milk, or both. In fact, a woman's lifestyle at any time between adolescence and menopause can critically affect her reproductive role and the nutrient requirements for properly fulfilling that role.

During infancy and childhood, boys and girls have essentially the same nutrient requirements. But girls bear the added burden of having to prepare for the years in which they will face the unique nutritional concerns of womanhood. With regard to this, only some of the specific nutrients that the body can store are of particular concern to women. Three such nutrients, all minerals, are crucial: iron, zinc and calcium. Two of them, iron and zinc, are often in short supply in the diets of infants and children.

But while boys will usually make up for a mild iron-zinc deficiency later in life, the reverse is true for girls: the demands of womanhood often perpetuate and aggravate this deficiency. Again, although calcium is almost never deficient in childhood, and in fact is deposited most rapidly in the bones (its primary storage site) during this period of life, many women will have lost enough calcium by their later years to cause serious problems. Consequently, the more calcium a young girl can get into her bones the better —and childhood may be the easiest time in which to accomplish this.

Childhood is also the period when, besides the body's storing certain nutrients, basic nutritional habits are formed. And since women are at greater risk than men for developing specific nutritional deficiencies, it is more important for a young girl than for a young boy to establish eating patterns that emphasize nutrient-rich foods.

In adolescence, the young girl experiences the fundamental changes that transform her into a woman. From the standpoint of nutrition, the most important of these changes occurs in the composition of the body's tissues. Both boys and girls begin with a similar body composition in which about 10 percent of the body weight is fat. But while boys retain this proportion of fat for the rest of their lives, girls undergo a change: By the time they become women, about 25 percent of their body weight will consist of fat. Too many calories, from any dietary source, will increase the already rapid rate of fat deposition that occurs in the body of the adolescent girl, and can result in obesity —a major problem among women of all ages and in all stages of development. Thus, the key to good nutrition for the adolescent girl is a diet that permits proper growth with enough fat to meet the body's needs while not leading to obesity.

For such reasons, good nutrition often seems to present

a paradox: How does one get enough of the nutrients such as zinc, iron and calcium that are needed for proper growth, with a little left over for the future, while at the same time not consuming too many calories? The simple guidelines in this book will ensure young girls of an adolescence that prepares them nutritionally for their adult years.

Good nutrition should also be part of the independent years that typically follow adolescence for the American woman. The dietary pattern most consistent with the lifestyle of today's woman is one of limited calories and foods having a high nutrient density. This requires concentrating on foods that are high in complex carbohydrates while avoiding those that are high in fat or refined sugar. The greater the variety of food choices in such a diet, the lower the risk of any nutrient deficiency.

Many young women experiment with different kinds of diets. Some try vegetarianism or some variation of it. This should not be a matter of concern: Most of the people in the world are modified vegetarians, and a vegetarian diet can be very healthful provided that it is not too restrictive and that some simple guidelines are followed.

But today's lifestyles often interfere with any type of diet a young woman may choose. Many of the oral contraceptives, for instance, obstruct the body's use of certain vitamins, while heavy alcohol consumption can limit the body's absorption of some vitamins.

Another important nutritional consideration for the young woman is in preparing for her first pregnancy and lactation. She should strive to be at the right weight for her height and to have built up adequate reserves of those nutrients that are particularly needed during pregnancy and lactation. This is one period in which special attention should be given to iron, zinc and calcium, which can be stored before pregnancy and are in short supply during that time.

All of the nutrients that the fetus needs for proper growth and development must be carried by the mother's blood to the placenta, and passed through that special organ into the blood of the fetus for transport to its tissues. Because this requires energy, women must consume more calories during pregnancy than they do before it. A woman of normal weight will have to gain at least twenty-five pounds during pregnancy, while one who is underweight will have to gain even more.

Some specific nutrients are also in short supply during pregnancy. Calcium, for example, is required for proper development of the fetal skeleton. Folic acid and zinc are needed for the rapid cell division that accompanies fetal growth and the formation of new red blood cells in the blood of both the mother and the fetus. However, the most important nutrient in short supply during pregnancy is iron.

In the case of men, iron can be efficiently stored in the body if its dietary intake exceeds its loss, and a boy who completes his adolescence with depleted iron stores can easily replenish these after his growth stops. The situation is quite different in young women, for whom it is very difficult to make up an iron deficit at the end of adolescence. Furthermore, when the young woman becomes pregnant, her deficit is likely to increase, with the cumulative effect being iron-deficiency anemia.

Moreover, because women normally consume less food and therefore considerably fewer calories per day than men, they receive a proportionately smaller amount of iron. For this reason, women must be much more concerned with a diet that emphasizes iron-rich foods. The recognition of the borderline amount of iron in the average

American woman's diet led to the iron fortification of many foods. Yet much of the iron in such foods was until recently in a poorly absorbable form. For the most part, this has now been corrected. Generally, about three times as much iron will be absorbed from such foods as meat and liver as from vegetable sources or fortified grains. For reasons like these, it is extremely important to prevent iron deficiency in the adolescent girl, and to supplement the diet with iron during pregnancy. In addition, women with heavy menstrual periods should either pay very careful attention to their dietary iron intake or should take a daily iron supplement.

Only half of all American women who give birth to babies nurse them. But whether you nurse or not, there are particular nutritional concerns that follow the birth of your baby. The nursing mother must avoid the nutritional deficiencies that can result from her infant's suckling at her breast. Here again, calcium is very important. Breast milk is high in calcium, which either is supplied by the mother's diet or is taken from her bones. All of the other minerals and vitamins are also required in greater amounts during nursing, so that the milk contains adequate supplies of them without the mother herself becoming depleted. Because the infant's total nutrition is coming from the mother's breast milk, even nutrients that are rarely deficient in men, women, or children can be deficient in a breast-fed infant. Vitamins B_{12} and B_6, for example, can be deficient in a breast-fed infant if the mother's supply is very low.

Vitamin B_{12}, like folic acid, is necessary for proper cell division and growth in an infant. But unlike folic acid, vitamin B_{12} is very abundant in the American food supply, being present in almost all meat and meat products, and can be stored by the body. Yet a deficiency of this vitamin (known as pernicious anemia) does occur when the supply is severely limited or the demand is particularly high, such as during a woman's reproductive years, or in the case of a woman who is a strict vegetarian. A woman who is both a vegetarian and is nursing may well have an infant that will develop a vitamin B_{12} deficiency unless measures are taken to prevent this.

Vitamin B_6 is necessary for proper functioning of the nervous system. Like vitamin B_{12}, it is widely available in our food supply, and as in the case of vitamin B_{12} men almost never develop a vitamin B_6 deficiency. Again, however, women require much more of this vitamin during pregnancy (when the fetus needs it for proper brain development), and can become at least mildly deficient in vitamin B_6 if their dietary supply is not increased during that time. Lactation, a particularly critical stage during the life cycle, also requires a greater intake of vitamin B_6. The young infant needs a great amount of this nutrient, and its mother's milk is the only available source. The mother's diet must therefore provide the vitamin for both her and her infant. Moreover, as with folic acid, both alcohol and oral contraceptives interfere with the absorption of vitamin B_6, and to some extent with that of vitamin B_{12}. Hence, women whose lifestyles include alcohol and contraceptive use are at risk for a vitamin B_6 deficiency. But since vitamin B_6 is available in the food supply, and since its requirement increases only during pregnancy and lactation, a vitamin B_6 deficiency is much rarer and usually milder than a deficiency of folic acid.

Perhaps the most important nutritional factor for the lactating mother is her calorie intake. She will require considerably more calories than she did before and even during pregnancy. If her weight is normal, this will present no problem; her appetite will increase naturally, and with it her food intake to compensate for the extra energy she expends in milk production. For an overweight woman, careful control of her food intake can allow her to lose weight without compromising her milk supply.

Women who do not choose to breast feed must still pay careful attention to their nutrition in the months following delivery. Unless they control their calories, they may retain the fat that their bodies collect in pregnancy for use during the lactation period. The weight gain many women experience after pregnancy may, in fact, be related to their not having nursed.

Because most of a woman's reproductive years are not occupied either by pregnancy or by lactation, there is usually ample time to for her to replenish her body's supplies of depleted nutrients between pregnancies and after her family has reached its final size. Yet even during these times, women continue to lose nutrients during their menstrual periods. These losses must be taken into account as a woman builds up her body's nutrient reserves.

During and after the childbearing years, the nutrients in greatest demand are iron, zinc and folic acid, all of which are needed to compensate for the blood that is lost during menstruation. At the same time, women must replace the calcium they may have lost during pregnancy and lactation, and make up for any loss of this nutrient before menopause occurs. It is also important for a woman to limit her calorie intake, since obesity often occurs during this time of life, presenting health risks with advancing age. Thus, while certain nutrients must be consumed in large amounts, calories must be controlled. This may seem like a contradiction, but it really isn't. As we shall see, the key to success is a diet of high nutrient density, with each calorie representing as many nutrients as possible.

Calories are present in all foods absorbed into the body, but the type of food that supplies them is critical. Some foods deliver high quantities of various vitamins and minerals along with their calories. These are the nutrient-dense foods. Other foods deliver very little besides calories. These are the nutrient-poor foods. Still other foods, such as pure refined sugar and certain types of alcoholic beverage, are devoid of any nutrients except calories. These have often been referred to as the "empty calorie" foods.

Thus, as a woman alternately increases and decreases her caloric intake, particularly when trying to lose weight, her intake of certain nutrients will also go up and down.

The importance of limiting calorie intake by limiting foods that have a low caloric density and encouraging foods that have a high caloric density becomes much greater during a woman's later reproductive years—the period when obesity becomes an increasingly serious problem, for with increased weight comes an increased risk for such diseases as atherosclerosis (hardening of the arteries), high blood pressure, diabetes, cancer of the uterus, gallbladder disease, and several others. But while reducing caloric intake is important to many women's health, these same women often require increased amounts of certain other nutrients. This can be accomplished, and as we shall see, isn't even really difficult.

Finally, women live longer than men: A newborn girl can expect to live eight years longer than a newborn boy, and women make up two-thirds of the elderly American population. In the total population sixty-five years or over in 1981, there were about 147 women for every 100 men. By age eighty-five and over, there were 224 women per 100 men. Because of their greater longevity any nutritional problems that plague women in their early years are likely to be exaggerated in later life. Among these are various vitamin and mineral deficiencies as well as certain nutritional problems that are common with increasing age generally, but occur much more often in women than in men. For example, some types of cancer in women are associated with long-term nutritional practices. The most prominent of these are cancer of the breast and uterus. Perhaps the most common nutrition-associated disease in older women is osteoporosis, which is both more common and more severe in older women than in older men. More than 20 percent of women over sixty-five suffer from this disease, which in its most severe form can lead to fractures of the hip or vertabrae (spinal bones). Such fractures are ten times more common in women than in men. We shall discuss the intake of calcium throughout a woman's lifetime as an important determinant of osteoporosis, and will review some exciting new research that is revealing the precise cause of and possible treatment for this illness.

One food substance that is extremely important for older people is actually not a nutrient—fiber. Fiber is a form of complex carbohydrate that is not broken down in the gastrointestinal tract, and is therefore not absorbed into the body. It supplies no calories, vitamins or minerals, although foods high in fiber may also be high in vitamins and minerals. As it passes through the gastrointestinal tract, undigested fiber traps many substances within its netlike structure. The most important of these is water, since this renders the stools softer, requiring the muscular walls of the bowel to generate less pressure in order to move the bowel contents along. As a result, the time during which waste products must remain in the gastrointestinal tract is reduced. Because constipation is a serious problem among the elderly, a diet high in fiber—for reasons such as these —will often bring relief. There is also some evidence that cancer of the colon may be less common in people who consume a high-fiber diet. Finally, a high-fiber diet can prevent or relieve the disease known as diverticulitis, which is quite common in older persons.

CHAPTER 2

The Very Young Child

*F*rom birth to the beginning of puberty, girls and boys grow at nearly the same rate. Boys may require somewhat more calories because of their generally greater activity, but even this has changed in recent years as girls have begun to lead much more active lives than they once did. Yet an even more abrupt change takes place when a girl enters adolescence, with her nutritional requirements becoming very different from those of boys, in preparation for young womanhood, childbearing and later life. Because of this, the nutritional practices of girls require special attention over and above those of boys.

Let us begin at birth. The best food for any newborn infant is breast milk. It is important because it contains calcium and phosphorus in the right ratio for promoting rapid calcium deposition in the bones—the ultimate storage depot for all of the body's calcium. Breast milk also contains iron and zinc in forms that the body can easily absorb, and hence will promote the storage of these nutrients in the nursing infant. Another important point is that breast-fed babies tend not to overeat as much as formula-fed ones, since they control their own intake and stop feeding when satisfied. By contrast, mothers will "stuff" the last ounce in from a bottle. Thus formula-fed babies accumulate more fat, an excess of which can be a particular liability to the young girl entering puberty. For one thing, girls are more prone than boys to obesity (too high a percentage of body fat) during the adolescent period. More important, however, is that women are more prone than men to obesity during adulthood, and fat children of either sex are very likely to become fat adults. This is because childhood obesity usually results from the development of too many fat cells in the body, a condition that once established is likely to remain throughout life. There is also some evidence that childhood obesity is associated with a slight but significant increase in the incidence of uterine cancer in adulthood.

Avoiding obesity means controlling calories and encouraging exercise. In children, the first warning of a weight problem is a weight gain that is out of proportion to an increase in height. Both a child's weight and height values can be plotted on graphs that serve as an "early warning" system for obesity.

After the nursing period, children derive their nutrients from a variety of foods. For girls, foods rich in the storable nutrients, of which calcium is probably the most important, deserve special attention. During childhood, the bodily machinery that promotes bone-calcium deposition is working at maximum efficiency, and the conditions for storing the maximum possible amount of calcium within the growing bones are ideal. Such perfect conditions will never again occur in a woman's life. Thus, while it may be difficult for the mother of a young girl to concern herself with her daughter's storage of calcium for a period fifty or more years in the future, this is the time for such concern.

What is necessary is to supply an adequate amount of dietary calcium. It is not necessary to go overboard, since the body will not absorb an excess of this nutrient. Adequate calcium can easily be supplied through dairy foods, green leafy vegetables and certain other foods. There is no need for calcium supplements. Yet it is not enough for the body to simply take in sufficient amounts of calcium; the conditions must be such that it is also absorbed as efficiently as possible. This means consuming enough vitamin D, which directly stimulates calcium absorption from food and calcium deposition from blood into bone. Vitamin D can be easily gotten from the diet, especially in dairy foods. Finally, favorable calcium absorption requires that the amount of phosphorus (another mineral) consumed at the same meal that provides the calcium must be kept low. For practical purposes, this means that a mother should not give her daughter foods that are high in phosphorus (red meats and certain carbonated soft drinks) at the same time as foods that are major calcium sources. A good rule to follow is to feed these different kinds of foods at least one hour apart.

Generally, iron and zinc come from the same foods: meat, eggs, green leafy vegetables, and in the case of zinc, seafood. Table 1 lists other foods rich in zinc.

Both iron and zinc are extremely important during growth, but once again, while emphasis must be put on providing enough of these nutrients in the diets of all children, girls—especially in the case of iron—merit special attention. Chronic iron deficiency is the most common nutritional problem in women. Moreover, at every phase in a woman's life cycle, her body makes special demands for iron. Once she "falls behind" in this nutrient, it is very difficult for her to catch up without direct supplementation. Therefore, a girl's body iron stores are more impor-

TABLE 1 ZINC CONTENT OF FOODS IN MILLIGRAMS (mg) PER SERVING

.2 TO .5 MG/SERVING		.5 TO 1 MG/SERVING	
egg	1 med.	puffed wheat	1 oz.
gefilte fish	3½ oz.	cheddar cheese	1 oz.
mango	½ med.	tuna	3 oz.
applesauce	1 cup	white rice	1 cup
pineapple juice	8 oz.	white bread	2 slices
tomato	1 med.	cranberry-apple drink	8 oz.
potato, cooked	1 med.	chicken breast	3 oz.
		milk (whole or skim)	8 oz.

1 TO 1.5 MG/SERVING		4 TO 5 MG/SERVING	
clams	3 oz.	beef (lean only)	3½ oz.
brown rice	1 cup	pork (lean only)	3½ oz.
whole wheat bread	2 slices	lamb (lean only)	3½ oz.
popcorn	2 cups	liver (beef and calf)	3 oz.
wheat germ	1 tbsp.		
bran (cooked, dried)	¾ cup		

OTHER	
9.4 mg—Pacific oysters (raw)	3½ oz.
74.7 mg—Atlantic oysters (raw)	3½ oz.

From: Nutrition and Health, *ed. M. Winick, Vol. 4, No. 1, 1982.*

tant than a boy's right from the beginning, and right from the beginning a mother should pay more attention to making sure her daughter's diet is one that is rich in iron. Table 2 gives a list of iron-rich foods that children like.

Because vitamin B_{12} is present in generous amounts in all animal products, most people do not have to worry about getting enough of it, and it is rarely deficient even in older women. But since this vitamin is required in greater amounts during certain periods of a woman's life, it is once again a good idea to build up the body's stores of it during childhood. Furthermore, many young women are vegetarians, and may have difficulty in meeting their vitamin B_{12} requirements—a problem that can lead to symptoms of

TABLE 2 IRON CONTENT OF FOODS IN MILLIGRAMS (mg) PER SERVING

.3–.7 MG/SERVING		.7–1.4 MG/SERVING	
fruits: e.g., apples, bananas, cherries, melons, citrus, pineapple, etc.	avg. size	rice, cooked (brown or white enriched)	1 cup
		tortilla (6 in. diam.)	1
corn grits	1 cup	cream of wheat	1 cup
popcorn (popped)	1 cup	wheatena	⅔ cup
bread (all varieties)	1 slice	wheat germ	1 tbsp.
enriched macaroni, spaghetti or noodles	½ cup	dry bulgur wheat	2 tbsp.
		pumpkin seeds	1–2 tbsp.
peanut butter	2 tbsp.	berries (all)	1 cup
mushrooms	⅓ cup	broccoli	1 cup
eggplant	½ cup	carrots	1 cup
tomato	1 small	collards	1 cup
		potato	1 med.

1.5–2 MG/SERVING		2–4 MG/SERVING	
barley	½ cup	amaranth	3½ oz.
buckwheat	½ cup	figs, dried	3 med.
oatmeal	1 cup	cooked peas & beans	½ cup
chicken (all cuts)	3–4 oz.	black strap molasses	1 tbsp.
bologna	3–4 oz.	tofu (soybean curd)	4 oz.
ham	2 oz.		
dried apricot halves	6 large		
green beans	1 cup		
brewer's yeast	1 tbsp.		

4–5 MG/SERVING	
beef (lean only), all cuts	3 oz.
lamb (lean only), all cuts	4 oz.
calf's liver	1 oz.
raisins	½ cup

From: Nutrition and Health, *ed. M. Winick, Vol. 4, No. 1, 1982.*

deficiency during pregnancy and at other times in a woman's life. One way to minimize this is to build up adequate stores of vitamin B_{12} during childhood.

During the past twenty years there has been considerable evidence that certain types of nutritional deficits in early childhood can have effects that last throughout life. Severe undernutrition during the first year of life, for example, can result in a permanent stunting of the brain size and in fewer cells and fewer connections between cells in the brain. But while the consequences of early nutritional deficit are largely the same in girls as in boys —with girls even being somewhat more resistant than boys to the effects of early undernutrition—one such early insult—exposure to excess dietary salt (sodium)—although affecting boys and girls equally, may have greater health consequences for girls.

Among Americans, blood pressure increases with age. Also, because women in our society live longer than men, the number of American women with high blood pressure is considerably greater than the number of men affected by this condition. Moreover, in some American population groups, such as among black persons, high blood pressure (hypertension) is more common in women of all age groups than in men.

In any population, hypertension is directly related to the consumption of sodium, mainly in the form of salt; the more salt consumed, the greater the incidence of hypertension. Furthermore, animal experiments have given evidence that a high salt intake early in life can result in hypertension later in life even with a low dietary salt content at that time. Thus, early exposure to salt seems to induce a susceptibility to hypertension that is not expressed for many years. It has also been shown that a preference for salt is a *learned* response, one that is often learned in infancy and childhood. The newborn infant will not seek salt, and if it is not supplied in large quantities in the infant's diet, will probably not develop a preference for it. Therefore, limiting an infant's or child's salt consumption may reduce its salt intake throughout life, with a proportionately decreased risk of high blood pressure—an outcome that would particularly benefit women. Baby food manufacturers, already under pressure to do so, have stopped adding salt to their products. It would be wise for mothers to continue this practice as their children begin to take table foods. Thus, if you must salt your food, it is best to do it out of your children's sight, and if you can limit the salt you add in cooking, both you and your children will benefit, with special benefits—as we have seen—for mothers and their daughters.

It is also very important for young children and particularly young girls, to have a diet that contains a wide variety of foods. Besides the calcium, iron and zinc derived from milk products, meats (including organ meats) and seafood, and the green leafy vegetables that are rich sources of many B vitamins, complex carbohydrates are also usually nutrient dense and provide fiber as well. There are no food groups that must be rigorously consumed. It is better for a mother to encourage her young daughter to try new things, developing as many tastes for as many different types of foods as possible. Then, as she begins her experience with food, you can simultaneously begin her experience with good nutrition. Helping your daughter to enjoy the taste of different types of foods will pay off in the long run, both positively and by preventing some of the nutritional deficiencies that are so prevalent in women from adolescence to old age.

CHAPTER 3

The Adolescent

*T*hroughout the animal kingdom, the process of sexual maturation brings profound change. Ugly caterpillars emerge from their cocoons as beautiful butterflies; aquatic tadpoles lose their tails, grow legs, exchange their gills for lungs and become air-breathing frogs and toads. Birds shed the dull plumage of their youth to emerge as brilliantly feathered adults. From the evolutionary standpoint, such changes are among the most important that an animal can undergo. They assure its ability to reproduce, and thereby the survival of its species. In a sense, human adolescence represents a similar metamorphosis.

In most mammals, and particularly humans, the changes of sexual maturation differ between males and females. Not only does this apply to the sexual organs, but also to body size and shape, the relative proportions of the internal organs, and the composition of various organs and tissues. The adolescent changes that result in a boy's becoming a man and a girl's becoming a woman are highly complex, involving both psychological and physical maturation.

Both sexes are affected by such internal factors as hormones and such external factors as nutrition. This chapter will deal with the special nutritional needs of adolescent girls and some nutritional problems common at this time of life.

PHYSICAL GROWTH

During adolescence, both boys and girls grow more rapidly than at any time since early infancy. The body weight nearly doubles, and almost 15 percent of the total adult height is added. Obviously this enormous increase in size in both sexes will require adequate nutrition if it is to occur smoothly.

Between the ages of three and ten, both boys and girls grow about two to three inches per year. The average girl begins her adolescent growth spurt just after age ten. Her growth rate rapidly increases, reaching a peak at around twelve years and gradually decreasing as she reaches full maturity. At the peak of the growth spurt some girls can add as many as four and a half to five inches of height in a year. The increase in body weight parallels that in height, in most girls following the growth in height by about six months.

In terms of adolescence, however, chronological age is a poor reference point, for while most girls will spend about five years of their lives as adolescents, the age at which a girl begins her growth spurt may vary from eight years in early maturing girls to almost fourteen years in those who mature very late. Thus, some girls can complete their adolescence before others even begin it. And since most of the physical and hormonal changes that characterize adolescence proceed in a fixed pattern once the process has begun, girls differing as much as six years in age can be in the same stage of adolescence.

Because of this marked variation in growth and development, adolescence, rather than being marked by age, is gauged physically by certain changes that occur as a girl becomes more mature. These physical changes are divided into five stages—the first being preadolescence and the last adulthood—on the basis of changes in the two sexual characteristics of pubic hair and breast development. The five stages are listed below.

TABLE 1

STAGE	PUBIC HAIR	BREASTS
1	Preadolescent	Preadolescent
2	Sparse, light colored, straight	Breast raised in a small mound; diameter of areola (brown pigmented area) increases
3	Darker, beginning to curl, increasing in amount	Breast and areola enlarge, no contour separation
4	Coarse, curly, abundant but less than in adult	Areola and nipple form secondary mound
5	Adult feminine triangle spread to inside of thighs	Mature; nipple projects, areola part of general breast contour

Changes in height, weight, body shape and the composition of organs and tissues are much better related to the five stages of maturity than to an adolescent girl's age. Similarly, an adolescent girl's nutritional requirements depend much more upon her stage of maturity than on her chronological age.

NUTRITIONAL REQUIREMENTS

The average girl will gain about forty-five pounds during the five years of adolescence. Almost twenty of these will be deposited as fat, with the remaining twenty-five pounds going into lean tissues, primarily muscle. By contrast, during the five-year adolescent period, the average boy will gain about fifty-seven pounds, only six and a half of which will be fat, with more than fifty pounds going into muscle and other lean tissues. Clearly, it takes a large increase in the quantity of almost all nutrients consumed by both sexes to achieve this major deposition of new body tissue. In fact, we can actually calculate the number of calories involved in the adolescent body-weight increase in both boys and girls. Going on the basis that protein provides about four calories per gram and fat about nine calories per gram, the adolescent girl has added 81,000 calories in fat and 48,000 calories in protein, a total of 129,000 calories in total deposited tissue. The adolescent boy has added 27,000 calories in fat and 92,000 calories in lean tissue for a total of 119,000 calories.*

THE NUMBER AND SOURCE OF CALORIES

We can see from the calculations above that girls consume slightly more calories during adolescence than do boys, even though girls gain less weight and fewer inches in height. This is not to say that boys require fewer calories during adolescence; boys actually consume a greater overall number of calories, but use them up, primarily through exercise, and also because of certain differences in metabolism. However, the high caloric intake that girls need for adequate growth is an important point to remember. Because the Food and Nutrition Board of the National Academy of Science sets the recommended dietary allowances (RDA) by age, they are only of general use during adolescence. However, while the RDA for girls aged 11 to 14 is

Protein = 1800 calories per pound or 112 calories per ounce.
Fat = 4000 calories per pound or 250 calories per ounce.

2,200 calories per day, with a decrease to 2,100 calories between the ages of 15 and 18, various studies have shown that many girls, despite consuming more than 2,500 calories per day at the time of their maximum growth (between stages two and three), do not deposit any excess fat. With increasing physical activity, which is certainly the social trend among girls, their caloric needs will approach those of boys. Moreover, because girls typically consume fewer calories than boys, they have a smaller margin of safety before their growth is compromised by a nutritional deficit. The adolescent girl who diets constantly may stunt her growth, particularly if she "crash" diets at a time when her growth rate is at a maximum.

Thus, the first nutritional rule to remember is that adolescent girls need more calories than adolescent boys. And how many more depends not on their age but on their stage of maturity, which will determine their growth rate.

Since girls deposit much less new protein in the form of muscle mass than boys, the increased demand for dietary protein that occurs during the adolescent growth spurt is much smaller in girls than in boys. Therefore, unless a girl is on a very restrictive diet, she should not have any problem in meeting the protein requirement. In fact, most Americans, male or female and in all age groups, consume far more than their RDA for protein. Also, because protein is available in a variety of foods including meats, fish, eggs, and dairy products, as well as in certain vegetables (particularly beans and grains), the adolescent girl can experiment with a number of eating patterns and still get plenty of dietary protein.

Similarly, she can derive the extra calories she requires from foods that will also supply generous amounts of vitamins and minerals. Such complex carbohydrates as whole grains and starches not only supply calories but also provide B-complex vitamins. Meat, besides being rich in protein, contains large amounts of readily available iron and zinc. Dairy products, also rich in protein, are good sources of calcium as well. And such natural sources of sugar as fruits, some vegetables and juices supply vitamins and minerals along with calories.

Although fats are concentrated sources of calories, the word on fat, given our present state of knowledge, is *moderation*. Unfortunately, however, many adolescent diets are particularly high in fat, and often in saturated (animal) fat. In our society, adolescents thrive on hamburgers and french fries, milk shakes and ice cream—all high-fat foods. And while it may not be dangerous for an adolescent girl to have a high-fat diet during the five years of her adolescence, since many of the fat calories will be used for growth and energy, it is important that a lifelong pattern of high fat consumption not be set at this time. On the other hand, because girls need more calories than boys during their adolescent growth spurt, they can safely consume more of these calories from non-protein sources. So, while a diet that consists solely of high-fat foods is inappropriate, a moderate fat intake means that an adolescent girl can "indulge" in some of the things that she likes without adversely affecting her health.

INCREASING BLOOD VOLUME

Besides bringing an increase in height and weight and a change in the body's tissue composition, adolescent growth also entails an enlargement of all of the body's organs. Since these organs must be supplied with adequate blood in order to function properly, the total volume of blood increases in both boys and girls during adolescence. Because of their greater growth, this increase is greater in boys. In girls, however, the need for an increasing amount of blood that begins during adolescence continues throughout the reproductive years. Part of this increased need for blood is due to the menarche, which begins at about the fourth stage of adolescence. In most girls this is about age fourteen or fifteen. With the beginning of the menarche, an ovum is released from the ovary each month and moves into the uterus, which is prepared to accept the egg only if it has been fertilized. The uterine preparation to receive a fertilized egg involves a major increase in the blood supply to the tissues of the uterus. If fertilization does not occur, the inside wall of the uterus is rapidly eroded and bleeds for several days in the process of menstruation.* In most women this regular monthly phenomenon continues until late middle age, and means a certain amount of chronic monthly blood loss that must be made up for by the manufacture of new blood.

Three nutrients are particularly important in the manufacture of new blood: the vitamins folic acid and B_{12}, and iron. Both folic acid and vitamin B_{12} are important in stimulating young red blood cells to divide and maintain a full blood cell supply. Iron is an integral part of hemoglobin, the pigment inside the red blood cells that carries oxygen to the tissues. Iron must therefore be present in sufficient quantity to provide normal quantities of hemoglobin within the red cells.

Despite the need for them, however, iron and folic acid are in marginal supply in the average American diet, and the dietary supply of vitamin B_{12} may be inadequate under certain circumstances (such as in strict vegetarians).

THE BLOOD-FORMING NUTRIENTS

Folic acid is required by all tissues for cell division. It is the vitamin in shortest supply in the average American

---

The cells of the inside lining of the uterus actually die because their blood supply is blocked and they fall away, leaving a denuded bleeding surface.

diet, and folic acid deficiency is the most widespread vitamin deficiency in the general population. This deficiency
is particularly prevalent during periods of rapid growth,
when the cells of the body's tissues divide most rapidly—
a situation that puts the adolescent especially at risk. Because overall growth, particularly muscle growth, is very
significant at this stage of life, folic acid deficiency can and
does occur, and attention should be given to foods that are
relatively high in folic acid, such as green leafy vegetables.

Two other vitamins often in short supply during adolescence are vitamins C and A. This situation occurs because
the kinds of foods adolescents favor are foods that contain
little of these vitamins, rather than because there is a short
supply of vitamin C- and A-containing foods available.
Simply increasing the dietary quantity of fruits and juices
will increase the vitamin C intake, while eating yellow
vegetables will do the same for vitamin A. Again, a variety
of foods will best ensure an adequate supply of these vitamins for the adolescent girl, and establishing such an eating
pattern in adolescence will protect her in the future, when
the requirements for various nutrients will increase.

The result of severe iron deficiency is anemia, a low
concentration of hemoglobin in the red blood cells. Studies
have shown that approximately 2.5 percent of all adolescent girls are anemic as a result of an inadequate body iron
supply. Although this may not seem like a very high percentage, it means that approximately one-quarter million
adolescent girls, of a total population of about ten million,
have iron deficiency anemia.

Perhaps even more significant is that some studies suggest that nearly 15 percent of adolescent girls—mainly girls
from lower socioeconomic groups and also those on reducing diets—have inadequate body iron stores and are therefore in danger of developing iron deficiency anemia. When
coupled with other studies suggesting that the average iron

intake among adolescents generally and adolescent girls particularly is below the recommended dietary allowance (RDA) of 18 mg per day, these findings establish the importance of increasing the dietary iron supply during adolescence. This increased iron intake is particularly important for girls, who will require an increased iron supply to meet their blood production needs for most of their lives. An iron deficiency during adolescence will be much more difficult for a girl to overcome later in life than for a boy.

Iron is present in foods of both animal and plant origin. However, only small amounts of the iron in food are actually absorbed into the body. The body has a special mechanism for conserving the iron within it and for preventing excess iron from being accumulated. This mechanism involves the reutilization of iron released from red blood cells when they "die" and the control of the amount of iron that is actively taken up by the cells in the gastrointestinal tract and moved into the body. Thus from 10 to 30 percent of the iron in meat (especially red meats and liver, as well as egg yolks and other animal products) may be absorbed, whereas only 5 percent may be absorbed from vegetable sources. The amount that is actually absorbed from either source depends on a number of factors, including the total amount of the food that is eaten, the form of the iron within the food, and the nature of the rest of the diet (for example, foods rich in vitamin C will increase iron absorption, whereas those that contain certain fibers will decrease absorption). Additionally, such factors as a person's age and the amount of iron already stored in the body are important in determining dietary iron absorption; adolescents absorb more iron than younger children or adults, while people with poor body iron stores absorb more than those with adequate stores.

Because of such factors, any recommendation for the amount of iron that should be consumed is highly individual, and the recommendations made for large groups of people, such as adolescent girls, are at best average approximations. The RDA of 18 mg per day of iron for adolescents assumes that about 10 percent will be absorbed—which, while probably reasonable for most adolescents, may not be reasonable for some. In order for absorption at this level to take place, at least some of the iron in the diet must come from meat sources, and adolescents who are strict vegetarians should therefore consume a greater total amount of iron-containing plant foods. Another, and growing source of dietary iron is iron-fortified foods. In the United States, such fortification is most common in breakfast cereals, from which the added iron is readily available and absorbed well (to about the extent to which vegetable iron is absorbed). Some cereals will supply the entire RDA for iron (18 mg) in a single serving. Most, however, supply about one-third of the RDA. There is no need to use cereal with the higher iron level if a balanced diet is being consumed, particularly if red meats are part of the diet.

Some people advise dietary iron supplementation—in the form of a tonic, a pill, or as part of a multivitamin-mineral preparation—during adolescence, particularly for girls. However, I see no need for this practice in the average adolescent girl, who with a little care should be able to get the iron she needs in her diet itself. Moreover, many iron rich foods will supply other necessary nutrients as well. Solving nutritional problems with a pill fosters poor eating habits, and should be discouraged, especially during the formative years of adolescence.

ZINC—A MINERAL WITH SPECIAL SIGNIFICANCE TO THE ADOLESCENT

Zinc is essential for many important body functions, including cell division and the synthesis of new protein.

The adequacy of this mineral in the American diet, particularly during periods of rapid growth, has stirred recent concern. The requirements for zinc during adolescence are less clearly defined than those for iron. However, overt zinc deficiency as a disease is particularly serious in adolescents, and reports of this deficiency from various countries have described poor development of the sexual organs and dwarfism in both boys and girls. Fortunately, such severe zinc deficiency does not occur in the United States. Nevertheless, zinc levels among certain groups of American adolescents, particularly those who are iron deficient, have been found to be somewhat low. Foods rich in zinc include meat, fish, poultry (particularly dark meat) and shellfish. When these sources are unavailable, legumes (peas and beans) are important sources of the mineral. The quantity of zinc in dairy products is relatively low. The best sources of zinc are therefore similar to those of iron, and the absorption of zinc, like that of iron, is better from meat than from plant sources. Because of these factors, the adolescent girl who eats iron-rich foods will also fulfill her zinc requirement.

The requirement for calcium is high in both girls and boys during adolescence since about 45 percent of the body's total skeletal mass is laid down during this time. In girls, both pregnancy and lactation will demand high quantities of calcium, and it is therefore fortunate that the absorption of calcium through the gastrointestinal tract is in both sexes highly efficient during adolescence (about twice as efficient as it will be later). The calcium deposited in the bones of the adolescent girl serves her current needs and is a stored source of this mineral for later needs.

The principles for maximizing calcium deposition in bone are the same for the adolescent girl as for the young child (see Chapter 2). First, the diet should contain an adequate amount of calcium (1,200 mg/day). Dairy products in the form of milk, cheese, yogurt and ice cream are all rich sources of calcium. Other, less well-known sources are the green leafy vegetables, which have the added advantage of being low in calories and fat. A "light" lunch consisting of a green salad and cottage cheese is rich in calcium. Second, the diet should contain enough vitamin D to aid in calcium absorption. Vitamin D "pushes" calcium from the G.I. tract into the blood and from the blood into the bones. The requirement is 400 I.U. per day. For most adolescents who consume dairy products or are exposed to the sun for moderate periods each day this is no problem, and vitamin D in the form of a dietary supplement is unnecessary and should be avoided. There is almost no circumstance beyond infancy when vitamin D supplementation is necessary. And too much D can be dangerous. Even strict vegetarians don't need vitamin D if they get enough sunlight. Third, a very high protein diet should be avoided, since an excess of protein over the dietary requirement increases calcium loss from the bones. (We don't know why this happens, but balance studies have shown that it does.) Fourth—as noted earlier—the phosphorus intake should be reduced when calcium is consumed.

Some of these recommendations may mean modifying the usual dietary patterns of adolescent girls. For example, a soft drink with a low phosphorus content is preferable to one that has a high content. When the label of such a beverage says "phosphate" or "phosphoric acid," the drink is high in phosphorus. If your adolescent insists on having that brand, see that she has it at least one hour after a meal that is supplying her with calcium. Skim milk is the perfect beverage from the standpoint of calcium absorption, but juice, tea, coffee or just plain water are much better than most of the carbonated soft drinks. Many of the dips found at parties are rich in calcium. Tell your daughter to try them (and remember this for yourself) with punch, juice or lemonade rather than soda. She or you may still feel guilty about the calories, but at least the calcium in them will be properly absorbed.

FOOD HABITS

During the preschool and early school years, a child's food habits are influenced mainly by family food choices, both at home and when the family goes out to eat. As a child reaches adolescence, however, other influences come to bear. Eating habits begin to be conditioned by the eating habits of friends and others who are not members of the family, and by the investment that food manufacturers and eating establishments put into their products through advertising and other promotions specifically aimed at teenagers. This is not to say that adolescents live in a world by themselves; they still live very much within the family and are still strongly influenced by how the family eats. Moreover, during this period, adolescents themselves can and often do affect the entire family's eating pattern. At least 65 percent of adolescent girls actively engage in shopping for and preparing the family's food. Adolescents also spend one out of every four dollars of the family's weekly food budget and many are rapidly becoming better informed consumers. Adolescent girls therefore have a significant influence on the variety of foods their families consume and on the brands used. But since adolescence is a time to try new things and growing numbers of adolescents are eating more of their meals away from the home, the local ice cream parlor has been widely replaced by the fast food chain as a place for adolescents to gather, and the eating pattern has generally changed from the ice cream soda after dinner to the hamburger and french fries, a pizza or a hero sandwich for dinner. Of course the pattern varies from one place to another. In an urban area or its suburbs, it may be easier for a youngster to break away from the family eating pattern than in a rural area. Still, in the United States today it is difficult to find any home so isolated that a McDonald's, a Burger King or a Pizza Hut is beyond reach. Yet such changing food habits are one form of the breaking away that is a natural part of adolescence, and in my judgment are not necessarily bad. They permit the adolescent to socialize over hamburgers, pizza, and soft drinks, which are far preferable to martinis, screwdrivers, and bloody Marys.

SNACKS

By their nature, adolescents are "now" people. They live for today with a feeling of immortality and indestructibility. For them, time is measured not in years or decades but in minutes, hours and weeks. These attitudes are carried over into their eating patterns. They are not concerned with the long-term consequences of fat and its association with heart disease or breast cancer later in life. They cannot think about salt and the high blood pressure or calcium and the brittle bones that may come later. These are light years away and of little importance to the adolescent concerned with looking her best for a particular social event, being accepted by her peers or winning the big race or tennis match. For the average adolescent girl, nutrition means satisfying her appetite while keeping her weight down, and supplying enough energy for her new, active lifestyle. Perhaps most important to her is that eating provides a vehicle for socializing with friends, away from the adults who previously ruled her life. With these short-term goals one might think that the average adolescent girl is slowly ruining her health with her eating habits. Nothing could be further from the truth.

For example, adolescents as a group skip very few meals

unless they are on some sort of diet, although they get only about 80 to 85 percent of their calories at meal time—the other 15 to 20 percent coming from snacks. However, many studies have shown that breaking up one's total food intake more evenly throughout the day is healthier than limiting it to three meals. Therefore, if snacking is part of a pattern of social rebellion (and I don't think it necessarily is), then the adolescent girl is replacing a standard eating pattern with a better one. Of course the kind of snack an adolescent girl eats is very important; if the snack contains only empty calories, it is unlikely that the remaining three meals can adequately supply the rest of the required nutrients, and a snacking pattern made up entirely of empty calories (calories with no other accompanying nutrients) should therefore be discouraged.

However, most studies of adolescent eating patterns have not found the horrible nutrient intake that we have been led to believe about the adolescent diet.

For example, several surveys have shown that 20 percent of the calories in the adolescent diet came from snacks, but that these snacks also delivered 12 percent of the protein, 20 percent of the calcium, 11 percent of the iron, 14 percent of the vitamin A, 13 percent of the thiamin (vitamin B_1), 17 percent of the riboflavin (vitamin B_3) and 18 percent of the vitamin C needed in the diet. As I pointed out earlier, the amounts of certain nutrients, such as iron, calcium and vitamin A, are low in the adolescent diet, but the proportion of these nutrients in snacks, when compared to the number of calories consumed in snacks, is remarkably good and suggests that the overall nutrient input that snacks contribute is proportionally similar to that contributed by the rest of the diet. Thus, rather than indicating that the adolescent girl mainly consumes empty calories when she snacks, the foregoing data indicate that she does much better than the adult population. And since snacking is meant to be fun, the adolescent girl does very well in getting some important nutrients in the form of snacks.

Furthermore, with certain minor changes, the snacks an adolescent girl consumes can not only be brought up to the nutritional standard of the usual family diet, but can even be used as specific sources of some important nutrients. With regard to this, parents should remember that it can be their attitude toward snacking generally and to their daughter's snacking pattern particularly that will determine whether she will be receptive to minor alterations in this pattern. It is best to start with a positive approach. By encouraging the eating of foods that many adolescents already like, such as cereals and bread, for example, and perhaps suggesting or supplying whole-grain or enriched products for this purpose, a mother can encourage her daughter to increase the nutrient density of a snack. Similarly, the substitution of fruit for candy or ice cream for potato chips will markedly increase the nutrient value of a snack. A supply of such nutritious snacks as fresh and dried fruits, nuts, whole grain crackers and cheese should also be kept on hand, and alternatives that fit into the adolescent's snacking pattern should be offered.

Above all, parents should not be rigid about a child's eating habits; there are many ways of increasing the value of snack foods, and even if a parent is not completely successful in improving an adolescent's eating habits, it is comforting to know that the eating pattern most adolescents have chosen for themselves is more nutritious than the pattern used by most adults.

FAST FOODS

A fine line sometimes exists between what constitutes a snack and what constitutes a meal in the overall eating pattern of the adolescent. With regard to this, the fast-food or "take-out" meal has several things to offer: the foods are inexpensive, yet safe and familiar; the items served are foods that adolescents like, and are available quickly at almost any time of the day or night. Also important—at least socially—is that the eating establishments are frequented by other adolescents. It thus seems that, at least for the foreseeable future, the fast food chains are with us, for better or for worse.

From the standpoint of nutrition, and particularly adolescent nutrition, what does this mean?

Unfortunately, there have been few systematic studies of the nutritional value of the meals served in different types of fast-food establishments. Most such eating places have only a limited number of items, and some individual items have been singled out as being low in certain types of nutrients. However, the combinations of these items that the patrons of fast-food establishments usually eat have not been carefully analyzed. McDonald's has had samples of its major food items directly analyzed, and claims that the combination of a Big Mac, a serving of french fried potatoes and a chocolate milk shake provides 40 percent of an adolescent's daily energy requirements and more than this percentage of protein, vitamin C, thiamin, riboflavin, niacin, calcium and iron. Only vitamin A is in short supply, comprising about 10 percent of the daily requirement. But while such figures may look good on the surface, the true value of the nutritional input in any fast-food meal depends on the combinations of foods selected. If the shake is replaced by a soft drink for instance, the number of calories will be fewer, but the calcium will be markedly reduced. The important thing for the adolescent girl is therefore to make the right fast-food choices in terms of those nutrients that she needs for growth and must store for the future.

Three major nutritional problems are common to many fast-food eating places: the foods they serve are often high in calories, high in fat—particularly saturated fat, and high in salt. Too many calories lead to obesity, which is a problem in adolescent girls;. a high intake of fat—as we have noted—may be associated with breast cancer in later life, and excess salt may result in high blood pressure, another problem with particular significance for women.

There are three ways of reducing the effects of these problems. The first is to patronize places serving foods that are lower in these substances; for example, pizza and spaghetti places. The second is to compensate in the rest of the diet by reducing the amount of salt and fat consumed at home. The third is to make choices with this problem in mind. For example, many fast-food places have instituted salad bars, and choosing a salad (without the creamy dressing) in place of french fries or ordering broiled instead of fried fish can cut down on both fat and salt. Avoiding pickles and relish will also cut down on salt.

One solution to the problem of fast foods, then, is for parents to encourage their children to frequent those places that serve the widest variety of foods, particularly foods low in fat and salt, and at the same time to have available at home, both at mealtimes and for snacks, foods low in fat and salt and high in some of the nutrients, such as vitamin A, that may be lacking in fast foods.

OBESITY

Generally, when a person's weight for a given height increases from 10 to 20 percent above the ideal weight for that height, the person is considered only mildly obese. More than a 20 percent increase means frank obesity. We have also already noted that adolescent girls deposit fat at a much more rapid rate than adolescent boys. Only recently, however, has it begun to be understood just how fat is deposited during this period in a woman's life.

Fat is contained within specialized cells called adipocytes, or fat cells. Each cell contains a globule of fat that takes up most of the space within the cell, pushing the other cellular elements aside. Each fat cell is also capable of enlarging to accommodate an increasing amount of fat as it accumulates. Thus for most people, particularly in adulthood, becoming fat means filling up existing fat cells with more fat, like filling a balloon. Conversely, weight loss entails a shrinking down in the amount of fat within the fat cells, letting the air out of the balloon.

However, the number of fat cells is also important in determining the total amount of fat in the body, and while adolescent girls who grow normally deposit fat in many normal-sized fat cells, the obese adolescent deposits her excess fat not only through the swelling of existing fat cells but also by producing more fat cells. She is apt to have too many fat cells. Since an individual is unable to appreciably increase or decrease the numbers of fat cells once adult life is reached, this difference has enormous implications for the future of the obese adolescent, since a person who achieves normal weight by dieting but whose body contains too many shrunken fat cells may at any time refill these cells and regain the weight.

Therefore, adolescent obesity, unless it is reversed, will invariably lead to adult obesity, and—more seriously—will lead to a variety of adult obesity that is very difficult and often impossible to treat successfully.

Before discussing the reasons for adolescent obesity and its prevention and treatment, it is important to understand that many adolescents, particularly adolescent girls, perceive themselves as obese when in fact they are not. Some studies have shown that as many as 50 percent of adolescent girls have made at least one attempt at weight reduction by dieting. On the other hand, by even the most generous reports, less than 15 percent of teenage girls are obese. Hence, hundreds of thousands of young girls are on reducing diets and—at least for health reasons—don't need to be.

Part of the fixation on weight and the constant concern with body image among adolescent girls is caused by the social pressure of a society that worships extreme thinness, particularly in women. Furthermore, the number of young girls who perceive themselves as fat increases with age, in contrast to boys, who begin to perceive themselves as thinner as they get older. How often have you seen a group of teenagers having cold drinks at a sporting event? The chances are that the boys are drinking regular soda while the girls are consuming no-cal soda. This pattern of constant dieting, or (and even worse) of alternating periods of dieting and overeating, can create serious nutritional problems. As we have seen, some nutrients are hard to obtain in adequate amounts even when enough calories are consumed; if the number of calories is restricted, deficiencies in iron, zinc, folic acid, calcium and vitamins A and C will be much more common.

Because true obesity is a serious problem in adolescent girls, while the mildly obese girl or the one who is depositing fat too quickly is more difficult to recognize, certain simple measurements can be very helpful. First, the increase in height and weight should be proportional as adolescence progresses. If a girl's weight increases disproportionately to her increase in height, she is becoming obese. (However, an extremely muscular adolescent girl may have an increased weight for her height and still not be obese.) There are tables that relate weight to height in different age groups. Second, there are some measurements simple enough to be done in a doctor's office that will actually indicate the amount of body fat. Small calipers have been developed that are used to measure the thickness of the fat layer in different areas of the body, and a simple measurement at the back of the upper arm can tell whether a teenage girl is too fat.

There are undoubtedly many reasons why certain adolescent girls become obese and others do not, a number of which remain unknown. Some simply consume too many calories. However, it would be an oversimplification to say that the major cause of adolescent obesity is caloric overconsumption alone, since many studies have shown that obese children do not necessarily consume more calories than their lean counterparts. In fact, they may actually consume fewer calories. Some people have said that an increased consumption of sweet foods is responsible for obesity in this age group. However, the evidence does not support this statement. Taste tests have shown that obese teenagers reject sweetened test preparations more than lean teenagers, and that after losing weight they have the same taste perception for sweets as adolescents who were never obese. Finally, it has been claimed that adolescents who are obese are much less active than those who are lean, and that even when engaged in sports they expend much less energy. But while there are studies that bear this out, it is difficult to say which came first, the obesity or the inactivity. Perhaps these children are inactive because they are obese rather than obese because they are inactive. Or perhaps both factors work together, producing a vicious cycle that favors the deposition of fat.

Whatever the reason for its occurrence, the problem of obesity in adolescent girls cannot be ignored, both for health and for social reasons. From the standpoint of health these teenagers are apt to continue their obesity into adult life and be endangered by the adult complications of obesity. From the social standpoint, obese people generally and obese adolescents especially meet discrimination under all kinds of circumstances. Other things being equal, the obese girl has a harder time getting into college or getting a job than her slimmer classmate; she may be the butt of cruel jokes by classmates and peers, and is usually the last to be asked to the prom or to other social events. This overt discrimination against obese youngsters is a kind of "health bigotry" that is difficult to understand, especially in an adolescent society that has become increasingly open and egalitarian. However, it often prompts the obese girl to withdraw and seek solace in food, even if she didn't overeat before. Society has made it difficult for her to accept her obesity and to deal with it.

Obesity is much easier to prevent than to cure, particularly in adolescent girls. Whatever the reason, it is the *rate* of weight gain that is important, and not the actual weight itself, since all adolescents must normally gain weight. For a girl who is gaining too much weight for her rate of growth, limiting the calorie intake may allow her to continue to gain weight more slowly while still growing properly, permitting her to "grow out" of her obesity. However, if there is too much control of her calorie intake, her growth may be stunted. For a girl in whom the first signs of overweight begin after the growth spurt, the calorie control may have to be greater; her weight may have to be maintained with no further gain while allowing an adequate calorie intake for the remainder of her normal growth. Obesity appearing at the end of adolescence should be managed in the same way as for an adult.

The success in controlling severe adolescent obesity, with the overweight teenager emerging from adolescence as a slim adult, is often not very good. The first and perhaps the most difficult thing that a very obese adolescent girl must accept is that she will probably have a weight problem for the rest of her life. The second thing that she must do is to set reasonable body-weight goals, and when she attains them, maintain them. A twelve-year old girl who is thirty pounds overweight before entering her growth spurt can, for example, set the following goals: twenty pounds overweight by the end of her growth spurt and ten pounds overweight by the end of adolescence. Such goals are attainable, and while this girl may never attain the slim image portrayed by the beauty magazines, she will have prevented some potentially serious weight-related health problems. If, on the other hand, she were to set the goal of losing her thirty pounds of excess weight during the next year, she would almost certainly fail, become frustrated, continue her poor eating habits and wind up with a serious obesity problem.

The principles governing weight loss in adolescents are the same as those in adults: More calories must be expended than are consumed. Obviously this can be attained by taking in fewer calories, burning up more calories, or both. In the mature woman, although increasing exercise will certainly help a weight-loss program, the main emphasis is on diet. In the adolescent girl more emphasis can be put on increasing activity; the more active the girl the less drastic the diet. During adolescence there are unlimited opportunities for burning off calories, including such sports and games as roller skating, bicycle riding, dancing and others. Even walking, since if adolescents returned to using their own power for getting from one place to another, the incidence of obesity in this age group might well begin to drop. Table 2 lists the number of calories expended during various activities.

A weight-loss diet for an adolescent girl should be planned and followed with great care. Fad diets and crash diets, which will be discussed in detail in Chapter 7, are particularly dangerous in adolescence. All such diets are inadequate in certain nutrients, and hence will induce nutrient deficiencies during this period of increased nutritional need. The best diet is one that limits calories and yet

TABLE 2 CALORIE EXPENDITURES PER HOUR FOR DIFFERENT ACTIVITIES*

ACTIVITY	CALORIES EXPENDED PER HOUR OF CONTINUOUS EXERCISE
Bicycle riding	200–600
Walking moderately fast	200–300
Football	560
Soccer	560
Frisbee	200
Basketball	500
Tennis	500–700
Volleyball	300
Swimming	300–600
Dancing	200–400
Jogging	400–500
Skiing (cross country)	650–1,000
(downhill)	350–500

*Based on an individual weighing approximately 130–150 lbs. Add on more calories if the person is heavier.

From: Nutrition and Health, ed. M. Winick, Vol. 2, No. 4, 1980.

contains all of the essential nutrients. Examples of such diets are given in Chapter 7. Moreover, even on a "good" reducing diet, the adolescent girl should take a vitamin and mineral supplement. Any of the standard daily supplements that contains the recommended daily allowances of vitamins and minerals is satisfactory for this purpose.

If you are an adolescent girl who needs to lose weight, remember that time is on your side. If you carefully reduce your caloric intake and increase your activity, you can modify your weight gain so as to allow the natural growth that accompanies adolescence to be your ally. Don't be in a hurry; set reasonable goals. Develop a plan of eating and activity and stick to it. Don't get discouraged if you do not attain instant success. Patience, one of the most important of all virtues, is a particular virtue when you are trying to lose weight.

SPORTS

Six million high-school students currently participate in interscholastic sports programs. Millions more take part in intramural team sports and in sports at the junior high school level. Furthermore, many communities sponsor activities such as dancing, swimming and gymnastics within their programs for teenagers. As a result, both the number of sports available to young people and the number of participating youngsters have increased dramatically. Furthermore, while only a generation ago most schools had no interscholastic sports for girls, up to 60 percent of teenage girls now spend some time in serious school athletic programs.

Partly as a result of this, growing numbers of world-class athletes are now in their teens, and sometimes in their early teens. Fifteen-year old girls reach the tennis finals at Wimbledon, make Olympic skating, swimming or gymnastic teams, or participate in world championship track and field or winter sports events. Even those who reach the top in their early twenties have spent most of their adolescent years in dedicated training. Today, the adolescent athlete —girls as well as boys—has become an important part of the "culture of youth."

When done appropriately, participation in sports can have a very positive influence on the adolescent. It builds security, fosters self-esteem and provides ego gratification through parent and peer approval. Beyond the character building aspects of sports lie the health aspects. The muscle work, exercise and expenditure of energy involved in regular athletic training increase vitality, foster feelings of well-being and contribute to the overall good health of the adolescent. Additionally, regular energy expenditure, especially by an adolescent girl, is the best possible insurance against obesity. On the other hand, if athletic participation is done inappropriately, with an adolescent being forced to take part against her will, or being constantly prodded to accomplish feats beyond her capacity, her self-image will be affected adversely.

One aspect of athletics is very important in the adolescent age group: Adolescent girls are very concerned about the changes in their bodies, and athletics gives them the chance to apply their bodies to new physical skills, often with the result of a better understanding of what the physical changes of adolescence mean in terms of strength and agility, as well as appearance.

Diet, of course, is a very important part of the athlete's life, and teenage athletes know this. They are concerned about the quantity and quality of the foods they eat—about such things as carbohydrates, fats, proteins, vitamins, minerals and fluids—concerns that the average adolescent does not share. Athletic participation has therefore created a large segment of the adolescent population that is intensely motivated to eat the proper foods.

During exercise, the body burns different kinds of fuel. If the exercise is moderate (walking rapidly for a short period of time), fat provides most of the energy. As the intensity and duration of the exercise increase, carbohydrates become the major fuel. At maximum capacity, carbohydrates become the exclusive source of energy.

Most of the energy used in sports that consume large amounts of energy, such as basketball, tennis, swimming and soccer, is supplied by glycogen—a carbohydrate that is stored in the liver and in the muscles. During prolonged exercise, the glycogen is converted into glucose, which circulates in the blood and is taken up by the tissues as their major source of fuel.

The body's capacity to store glycogen is limited, and during extended exercise, the amount of glycogen stored in the muscle becomes an important factor. For one thing, girls, because they have much less muscle tissue, can store much less glycogen than boys. For this reason their reserve energy capacity for sustained athletic performance is less than that of boys, and this is particularly true in girls who are smaller and have relatively less muscle tissue. In the active adolescent girl, these stores must therefore be replenished at regular intervals through the diet. A pattern of three meals and two snacks a day, with appropriate foods at these times, will replenish the amount of stored glycogen much more efficiently than will a big meal at dinner, snacking throughout the evening and eating irregularly during the rest of the day, particularly for the girl who must participate in late afternoon practice sessions. In girls, less than a thousand calories of energy are usually stored as tissue glycogen, and if these are replenished late in the evening they will be exhausted by midafternoon unless more food is consumed during the intervening daytime hours.

During each day, then, not only must enough calories be consumed to supply the energy for the next day's activities, but these calories must be consumed over an interval that will give the athletic girl her maximum reserves at the time her peak performance is demanded. Moreover, the calories consumed must be sufficient not only for supporting her normal growth, but also for maintaining her desired competing weight throughout the season of the sport in which she participates. The serious young athlete should therefore weigh herself at regular intervals. Often the coach or trainer will do this. A girl who is losing weight involuntarily is expending more calories than she is taking in, and her caloric intake should be increased. The best way in which to do this is to increase her consumption of high-nutrient-density foods.

To avoid the depletion of carbohydrate stores during

intense exercise, many athletes use what is commonly referred to as a carbohydrate-loading or glycogen-loading diet. The theory (not actually proven) is that glycogen stores can be raised and performance can be improved by removing dietary carbohydrate for a period and then reintroducing it at a very high level, "packing" the muscles with glycogen just before the competition. If there is a serious young athlete in your family, she will no doubt walk in one day and announce that with the big race or event only a week away, she is going on this diet. It is therefore important that both you and your youngster understand the principles of what she is doing.

In persons training for a marathon race, the diet is usually preceded by emptying the liver and muscle of their glycogen stores by running ten to fifteen miles at near maximum effort during the six days before the marathon. Similar depletion exercises are undertaken in other sports. After this the athlete lives on a carbohydrate-free, high-protein, high-fat diet for the next three days while continuing to train. This regimen will further deplete the muscle glycogen stores; however, it often leads to feelings of fatigue, a short temper, and lightheadedness, all symptoms of carbohydrate depletion, which may come on more rapidly and may be more severe in young women than in young men because their glycogen reserves are more easily depleted. During the three days before the race, the athlete then eats a high carbohydrate diet, often consisting of pasta, cereal and bread, building up the glycogen content of the muscles beyond its normal level.

I do not recommend this diet even for serious athletes. (In fact most world-class athletes no longer use it.) In women it can be particularly dangerous, since the timing for the carbohydrate depletion and repletion has been worked out on male athletes, and is probably quite different for women athletes since women have less glycogen and more fat in their bodies.

A much better approach is simply to go on a diet that has a high content of complex carbohydrates several days before the event. This will avoid the symptoms of depletion while still resulting in high glycogen levels before the competition.

An adolescent athletic girl who is concerned about not eating the proper foods may wish to record what she is eating over several days and, using some simple reference, such as the tables in this book, check that she is taking a diet varied enough to fulfill her daily requirements of the various nutrients. With this, she can be assured that her diet is supplying all of the essential nutrients.

Vitamin, mineral and protein supplements will not improve a person's athletic performance. They are also often expensive, and some are potentially dangerous. The only nutritional supplement that may be appropriate for a young woman participating in competitive athletics is iron. From 10 to 20 percent of menstruating women in the United States have low iron stores, and may therefore benefit from iron supplementation. Also, recent studies have shown that young women athletes with low iron stores, even if they are not anemic, will not perform as well as they should, and that simply supplementing their diets with iron can rapidly improve their performance. (It should be mentioned here that many young women athletes may cease to menstruate while training or competing regularly. There is no cause for concern if this occurs, since regular periods will resume as soon as the vigorous exercise is reduced. Such women, of course, will have a somewhat reduced need for dietary or supplemental iron.)

A specific body composition, in terms of the amount of body fat, is optimal for different types of sports. Because

TABLE 3   **RELATIVE BODY FAT VALUES FOR MALES AND FEMALES IN VARIOUS SPORTS***

SPORT	MALES FAT %	FEMALES FAT %
Baseball/Softball	12–14	16–26
Basketball	7–10	16–27
Football	8–18	—
Gymnastics	4–6	9–15
Ice Hockey	13–15	—
Jockeys	12–15	—
Skiing	7–14	18–20
Soccer	9–12	—
Speed Skating	10–12	—
Swimming	5–10	14–26
Track and Field		
Sprinters	6–9	8–20
Middle Distance Runners	6–12	8–16
Distance Runners	4–8	6–12
Discus	14–18	16–24
Shot Put	14–18	20–30
Jumpers and Hurdlers	6–9	8–16
Tennis	14–16	18–22
Volleyball	8–14	16–26
Weightlifting	8–16	—
Wrestling	4–12	—

*The values represent the range of means reported in various published and unpublished studies.

excess body fat reduces speed and quickness, limits endurance and contributes nothing to strength, the ideal for maximum athletic performance is to reduce one's body fat to the minimum compatible with fitness. However, the normally lower percentage of body fat in males than in females also applies to athletes. Simply stated, this means that a girl who participates regularly in any given sport should be fatter than a boy who participates in it. Table 3 lists the percentage of body fat that has been associated with top performance in a number of sports for both girls and boys. Since in mid-adolescence the average girl will have increased her percentage of body fat to about 15 to 20 percent, she will be normally at the desired composition at that time. Later she will have too much body fat and may need to diet. For certain sports, such as gymnastics and distance running, some weight control may be necessary. The fact that the optimal percentage of fat recommended for girls in many sports is the same amount of fat that a mid-adolescent girl normally has may partly explain the enormous success of many adolescent girls in athletics.

If an athlete must reduce the amount of fat in her body, a well-planned program of calorie control, which also meets all of the energy needs of her training, should be instituted. The first step is to determine the amount of fat to be lost by determining the existing amount of body fat (which is usually done by using the skin caliper measurement mentioned earlier) and projecting the optimal amount of fat desired for a specific sport (using Table 3). The rate of weight loss should be no more than two pounds per week. This can be done by creating a negative energy balance of about one thousand calories per day, partly through increased exercise and partly through reducing the caloric intake. Even when reducing to reach a desired fat level the athlete should not consume fewer than 2,000 calories per day. Crash dieting should never be undertaken for the purpose of attaining a desired weight. The adolescent who does this will weaken herself and perform poorly.

For the purpose of illustrating a fat-loss program, let us assume that a young woman weighs 120 pounds and that 25 percent of her body weight is fat. Thus, 30 pounds of her weight is made up of fat tissue. She wishes to attain an optimal body fat content for swimming, somewhere around 20 percent, or about twenty-four pounds of body fat. Her goal is therefore to lose about six pounds. She can do this over three to four weeks in the manner outlined above and still be able to consume adequate amounts of calories to perform well during this period. After she reaches her desired weight she can increase her caloric intake to achieve a balance.

Because of their concern over body fat, many young women athletes become overzealous in trying to reduce, often overestimating the amount of fat to be lost by harboring the erroneous idea that the leaner the better. Many also try to lose weight too quickly. Some of these young women develop a specific complex of symptoms that can ruin their athletic career and endanger their health. The syndrome is marked by a sudden aversion to food and a precipitous weight loss, including a rapid loss of body fat, muscle wasting and, in girls, an abrupt cessation of menstruation. Vomiting may result if the girl is prodded into eating, and the aversion to food will lead to problems of starvation. Athletes call this "flipping." Since the condition often occurs in a team setting, it is usually recognized in an early stage by teammates and coaches as the affected individual's athletic performance declines. Because of this, and with the help of sympathetic teammates and coaches who can offer support, the condition can generally be reversed and the symptoms will disappear slowly, allowing the athlete to continue to compete.

The energy requirements for such short term events as sprints, gymnastics, the pole vault or long jump can easily be maintained by consuming fluids regularly and eating small meals with a high carbohydrate content during the competition period. The fluids are important because an athlete will perform well only if her tissues are well hydrated. The fluid needs, including those for the replacement of sweat losses, are best satisfied with plain, clean, cool water. The minerals lost in the sweat—and especially salt—are easily replaced in the diet, since the sweating athlete is losing much more water than salt. In fact, beverages that have a high content of salt and other minerals, or the use of salt tablets, may worsen the dehydration. Additionally, the sugar and minerals contained in some "athletic beverages" are unnecessary for the well-nourished athlete, and reduce the feeling of thirst before enough water is consumed.

Planning for a proper food and fluid intake becomes more important in preparing for contests that last longer and require a more intense energy expenditure. The running games, such as basketball, tennis, and soccer, as well as sports such as rowing all demand a concentrated expenditure of energy over a relatively long period. For three to four days prior to competition in these sports, participants should have a diet that is high in carbohydrate, low in residue (bulk) and without high quantities of salt.

CHAPTER *4*

The Young Adult

Although the nutritional requirements of adolescent girls differ from those of boys, deficiencies can and do occur in both sexes. Furthermore, the nutrient requirements of the two sexes diverge even more after adolescence. Women must take in more of certain vitamins and minerals, and must accomplish this while controlling their calories by taking in less food. Men are in less need of these nutrients and can take in more food to meet their requirements. Consequently, women face the nutritional paradox of a constant battle to get more nutrients from less food. This chapter will present some simple guidelines for dealing with this paradox.

Fortunately, many young women are becoming more concerned with their health and with good nutrition. Often, the concern over weight, so pervasive in adolescence, carries into adulthood in the form of a much wider attentiveness than the adolescent fixation on body image. The young woman cares about fitness. Her new lifestyle stresses this, and many of her decisions about food are made in terms of it. She prefers not only foods that will keep her slim and fit, but also those that allow her to participate actively in all of the new and exciting things that are happening around her. If she can accomplish this she will resolve the nutritional paradox of being a woman.

A DIETARY PATTERN FOR FITNESS

There is no such thing as a "fitness" diet. However, there are ways in which a young woman can develop an eating pattern that will keep calories relatively low while at the same time offering variety in her foods and assuring adequate amounts of all the necessary nutrients for maintaining excellent health. Unfortunately, overweight is a chronic problem among many American women, and many young women who are not overweight wish to avoid gaining weight and choose to do this in a variety of ways. As a result, calories are often controlled by crash dieting or by starving one day and feasting the next, neither of which is satisfactory because they repeatedly shortchange the body of essential nutrients for brief periods of time. A diet plan that will truly reduce calories while supplying adequate nutrients is one that must be followed over a long time. Naturally, in any diet plan, there will be day-to-day fluctuations, but in a satisfactory diet plan the body will be able to cope with these. Remember, we are talking about a dietary pattern, not a method of dieting.

Since calories are the key to both weight loss and the maintenance of normal weight, let us begin with them. There are three sources of calories in the foods that we eat: fat, protein and carbohydrate (alcohol is considered a carbohydrate). Every gram of fat can be converted into nine calories. Every gram of protein or carbohydrate can be converted into four calories. Every cubic centimeter of alcohol can be converted into seven calories. Each of these substances can be burned as fuel or converted to fat that is stored in the body as fat tissue.

Clearly, if we simply wish to cut calories, the most efficient way to do this is to cut the amount of fat in our diets. And since the American diet is too high in fat and too much fat offers specific risks for women, the first rule in a dietary plan for fitness is to reduce the amount of fat consumed. But before we cut any calories from our diet, we should consider that maximum fitness requires adequate amounts of every noncaloric nutrient, including all of the vitamins and minerals. Therefore, the foods that we consume should contain the greatest possible concentration of noncaloric nutrients. Thus, the second rule in a dietary plan for fitness is to minimize our consumption of alcohol and of foods that contain large amounts of refined sugar—the two major "empty" calorie foods that deliver few if any of the necessary vitamins and minerals. There may be no problem when an athlete consuming 3,500 calories a day takes in some empty calories while still getting adequate amounts of the other nutrients, but a young woman who limits her calories to 2,000 or 1,800 per day will find it much more difficult to get the required amounts of the other nutrients she needs. Therefore, the third rule in a dietary plan for fitness is to emphasize foods that have a high nutrient density. Since snacking is common to the busy schedules of many young women—as well as being a potentially healthy way of balancing the daily nutrient intake—Table 1 gives examples of some high- and low-nutrient-density snack foods. Notice that the nutrient density of some of the foods in the table can be increased in a relatively simple manner. For example, whole milk is an excellent food that provides a variety of essential nutrients, but almost all of these are carried in the nonfat part of the milk. Therefore, removing all or part of the fat converts milk into a much higher nutrient-density food.

TABLE 1 **HIGH- AND LOW-NUTRIENT-DENSITY SNACK FOODS**

HIGH NUTRIENT DENSITY	LOW NUTRIENT DENSITY
Low-fat milk	Whole milk
Dried fruit	Hard candy
Peanuts in the shells	Candy coated peanuts
Plain popcorn	Caramel corn
Orange juice	Orange drink
Apple	Apple danish
Pizza	French fries
Peanut butter on crackers	Sandwich cookies
Cheese and crackers	Shortbread cookies
Frozen yogurt	Ice cream pop

How does a young woman, concerned with her weight and fitness, use the three dietary rules to create an effective and convenient dietary plan that can be easily followed and maintained indefinitely? It really isn't very difficult. She must first decide approximately how many calories she will consume each day. This will vary from one woman to another, depending on height, body build and the woman's individual metabolism. A good starting point would be 2,000 calories. If this keeps her weight constant, she should maintain her intake at this level; if not, she should cut back to 1,900 or 1,800 calories a day. Once she has decided upon the number of calories that will maintain her weight, she must distribute them over the day in accordance with her lifestyle and a healthy eating pattern. For example, a young woman attending college may prefer a small breakfast and lunch, a four o'clock snack when her classes are done, a relatively large dinner and a snack at about ten o'clock during a study break. By contrast, a working woman may prefer a small breakfast, a morning coffee break, a light lunch, an afternoon snack and a fuller, more leisurely dinner. On weekends both may have a relatively large "brunch" and a full dinner with no snacks in between. Whatever the pattern, it can be accommodated by dividing the total daily calorie intake appropriately.

Let us take the eating pattern of the college girl above and work out a typical 1,800 calorie-per-day diet. A 300-calorie breakfast might consist of cereal and skimmed milk (150 calories), orange juice (60 calories), and toast and margarine (90 calories) with tea or coffee. Lunch might be a sandwich or a salad, yogurt and fruit (a total of approximately 300 calories), a four o'clock piece of fruit, a glass of milk with crackers or biscuits or tea or coffee with a small sandwich (about 150 to 200 calories). Dinner might consist of meat, fish or poultry, vegetables, rice or potatoes, salad, fruit and a beverage (about 900 calories). A ten o'clock snack might again be fruit or a beverage with crackers or biscuits (150 calories). So far as the total number of calories is concerned, the combinations are almost limitless. But since 1,800 calories will permit consuming much more food if it is low-fat food, low-fat dairy products and lean cuts of meat should be emphasized in the diet.

The second part of developing this dietary plan is to choose foods that have the greatest nutrient density. Here we want to be selective so that we can assure an adequate supply of the nutrients that tend to be short in women's diets. Let us illustrate this with the example of three hypothetical breakfast cereals. The important ingredients, as listed on the package, are shown below.

TABLE 2

	CEREAL A	CEREAL B	CEREAL C
Calories (per serving)	120	90	110
Thiamine (% RDA)	25	50	10
Riboflavin	25	50	10
Vitamin B_6	25	50	10
Vitamin B_{12}	10	10	10
Folic Acid	15	15	30
Iron	15	15	45
Zinc	—	—	25

From the standpoint of total nutrient density, cereal B may appear to be best; it is lowest in calories and contains a higher density of many of the essential nutrients. However, cereal C is the one that contains the highest density of those vitamins and minerals in shortest supply—folic acid, iron and zinc. Thus, if the rest of the diet is low in these nutrients, such as when very little red meat is consumed, cereal C might be the best choice. The use of low-fat milk with any of the three cereals will bring up the calories only moderately (to about 170) while supplying calcium, protein and other essential nutrients. Adding sugar will also increase the calories but provide no other nutrients, and will therefore decrease the overall nutrient density.

The three cereals given above are examples of fortified foods—foods to which nutrients have been added. The only vitamins and minerals in them are put there by the manufacturer. The advantage of using foods that have a naturally high nutrient density is that they are not only rich in the known nutrients, but will also probably be rich in nutrients whose requirements may not yet be known. Table 3 is a list of all of the known nutrients and their recommended daily allowances for adult women. It lists foods that contain each of the known nutrients in high density. It shows that there is a certain nutrient pattern among various food families. For example, B vitamins are found in whole grains; iron and zinc in meats, egg yolks and certain vegetables; folic acid in green, leafy vegetables; vitamin A in yellow vegetables; vitamin B_{12} in meat and dairy products; vitamin C in citrus fruits; and calcium in dairy products.

Use of the table permits the construction of a nutritious diet with considerable variety. This diet does not require a specific number of foods from one group or another, as some diets do. Nor does it use the concept of the four food groups. Rather, it permits variety while ensuring an ade-

TABLE 3   NUTRIENT REQUIREMENTS FOR ADULT
            WOMEN

NUTRIENT	REQUIREMENT (DAILY)	FOOD SOURCES
Protein	44 grams	Meat, dairy products, fish, beans, certain nuts, grains when properly mixed
Vitamin A	800 micrograms (4,000 I.U.)*	Liver, butter and margarine, egg yolks, leafy green vegetables, yellow/orange vegetables and fruits
Vitamin D	5 micrograms (400 I.U.)	Milk and other dairy products, exposure to sunlight, fish liver oils, salmon, sardines
Vitamin E	8 milligrams	Whole grains, vegetable and seed oils, green leafy vegetables, legumes and nuts, lesser amounts from meat, fish, dairy products and fruits
Vitamin C	80 milligrams	Citrus fruits and juices, cantaloupe, potato, tomatoes, strawberries, broccoli, cabbage, green peppers
Thiamin	1 milligram	Whole grain and enriched products, legumes, liver, pork, nuts, leafy green vegetables
Riboflavin	1.2 milligrams	Meat (including liver), fish, dairy products, enriched grains, fortified cereals, green vegetables and yeast
Niacin	13 milligrams	Liver, meat, whole grain and enriched products, legumes, nuts, yeast
Vitamin B_6	2 milligrams	Liver, meats, fish, whole grain and enriched cereals, grains, soybean flour, peanuts, yeast
Folic Acid	400 micrograms	Green leafy vegetables, liver, orange juice, other fruits, yeast, whole grains
Vitamin B_{12}	3 micrograms	Liver, meat, fish, dairy products, organ meats, tempeh
Calcium	800 milligrams	Dairy products, green leafy vegetables, almonds, clams, oysters (See table page 81 for detailed listing)

*International Units.

NUTRIENT	REQUIREMENT (DAILY)	FOOD SOURCES
Phosphorus	800 milligrams	Meat, soft drinks, dairy products, nuts, legumes, whole grains
Magnesium	300 milligrams	Whole grains, legumes, nuts, leafy green vegetables
Iron	18 milligrams	Red meat, liver, raisins (See table page 23 for detailed listing)
Zinc	15 milligrams	Seafood, meat, liver (See Table 1, page 22 for detailed listing)
Iodine	150 micrograms	Seafood, fish, iodized salt

quate supply of all of the necessary nutrients. Unlike many "diet plans," it also allows choice, a very important ingredient for a young woman beginning her independent existence. And once a dietary pattern that emphasizes enjoyable foods that are low in calories and high in nutrient density has been developed, use of the table will no longer be necessary.

There are two further points that a young woman adopting this kind of dietary pattern should remember. The first involves protein, which—besides providing calories—is made up of many small components called amino acids. Most of these amino acids can be synthesized by the body (mainly in the liver). However, eight of the amino acids cannot be synthesized and must be supplied in the diet for the body to be able to build its own protein-containing tissues. If all of these eight "essential" amino acids are present in the diet, the body's protein intake is complete. Meat, fish, dairy products and certain beans and legumes are complete proteins in that they contain the essential as well as the other amino acids. The average American woman will probably get adequate quantities of the essential amino acids if she consumes even small amounts of the foods just named. However, vegetarians must take certain precautions, discussed later in this chapter, to ensure an adequate supply of these amino acids in their diet.

It is important to remember that protein is useful to the body only if it is first broken down into its constituent amino acids (which happens in digestion), which are only then available for the body's use in building its own proteins: Eating gelatin (a very incomplete protein) will not deposit gelatin in your nails, and smearing protein on your head will have no effect on the protein structure of your hair or scalp.

The second important point for a young woman planning a diet involves fat, which, like protein, is also made up of smaller constituents, in this case known as fatty acids. At least one such fatty acid (linoleic acid) cannot be synthesized by the body and must therefore be supplied in the diet. Practically speaking, this represents no problem for a healthy woman no matter how little fat she consumes. There will always be enough to supply the very small quantities of essential fatty acids that the body needs.

Whether you are a young college student, an aspiring young executive responsible for your own health or a young woman setting up a household, and are concerned with weight and with fitness, the eating program outlined above will prove worthwhile; it approaches the dietary guidelines recommended for all Americans, emphasizes slimness while offering a free choice and a wide variety of foods and ensures that the body will get adequate amounts of all the nutrients it needs.

COMMON DIETARY PITFALLS

A number of common situations in the active lifestyle of many young women are pitfalls to remaining on a dietary program aimed at fitness. Parties, whether in the office or social events, can be one such pitfall. The universal "coffee break" at the office is another. So is the lunch with a client. All of these situations can be kept under control with the use of a little restraint and preplanning.

The major problems at all parties are the drinks and hors d'oeuvres. Alcohol, as we have already noted, is almost totally devoid of all nutrients except calories. Furthermore, excessive quantities of alcohol can interfere with the absorption of certain nutrients. However, wine, besides having calories, may also have small amounts of some nutrients, and is therefore preferable to a cocktail if the choice has to be made. You can calculate your wine calories into the total calories for the day of a party or dinner at a restaurant by eliminating the midafternoon or late evening snack for that day.

Soft drinks are another significant source of calories unless they are artificially sweetened. The calories in these beverages are in the form of refined sugar, and hence their nutrient density is very low. Some soft drinks are also high in phosphorus, which interferes with calcium absorption. Orange juice or fruit punch is therefore much preferable to soda pop as a beverage.

Even more dangerous than the liquid refreshments at a party may be the hors d'oeuvres. Cold cuts are high in fat, as are cocktail frankfurters and meatballs. Anything fried is also high in fat, and some cheese spreads contain lots of calories. Also, beware of the dips. The creamy kind are often high in both calories and fat. Use them sparingly. By contrast, shrimp with cocktail sauce, crabmeat or other types of seafood are good dietary choices, and raw vegetables, which are becoming increasingly popular as a party food, are extremely nutrient dense.

The trick is to be aware of what you choose. When someone comes around with the platter, choose; don't grab. After a while the right choices will become automatic.

Lunch with a client may be an important business event and you may want to do things a little more festively than usual (especially if the company is paying). There is no reason why you can't do this and still stay on your fitness program. On the day of your luncheon, exchange the calories to be consumed with those you would ordinarily consume at dinner. Instead of having two martinis (300 calories), have one glass of white wine (100 calories) or a kir (125 calories). From there things are relatively simple. Choose foods of high nutrient density and keep the fat down. Avoid the bread or rolls and butter, the french fried potatoes, the creamy salad dressing and the sour cream on your baked potato, and don't order a main dish drenched in a heavy gravy. Just as with a party, the rules are the same as at other times, even though the temptations are greater.

As for those coffee breaks, stay away from the donuts and Danish pastries; they supply lots of calories and few other nutrients. Other types of cake, whole-grain cookies, or cheese and crackers are better choices. As for the coffee itself, those teaspoons of sugar add up. Besides, caffeine is a definite stimulant that may be useful in the short run but can produce a letdown later on. Finally, coffee—decaffeinated or not—causes heartburn in some people. Other pitfalls to a dietary program may be television viewing, which is a time of unconscious eating for some people, and studying for exams, which often leads to eating from anxiety. It is important that you be aware of your own pitfall situations and take measures to avoid them.

CONVENIENCE

Our modern food supply depends on a certain amount of processing to prevent spoilage, to extend the shelf life of a particular product, to put back or "improve" on nature's taste and to assure a constant flow of seasonal foods transported over sometimes great distances. This processing may remove some nutrients and add others, some of which are desirable and some of which are not. Freezing, for example, generally preserves the nutrient content of a food better than canning. Many processed foods also contain non-nutrient additives for keeping the foods fresh or for flavoring or color. Fortified foods contain nutrients (usually vitamins and minerals) that have been added in specific amounts; some of the nutrients provided in this way are in short supply in the human diet, and their addition therefore serves a useful purpose. Other fortified foods simply contain nutrients in numbers and amounts that make them sound better than their competitors in a television commercial.

The matter is not one of whether processed foods themselves are good or bad. It is simply one of choice. You can choose a processed food that is relatively low in calories and yet provides generous amounts of nutrients usually lacking in the American diet, such as a breakfast cereal fortified with folic acid, or you can choose a processed food that may offer better overall nutrition than the original, such as low-fat milk or yogurt—both choices which are nutritionally sound and convenient—or you can make a poor choice, such as heavily salted potato chips, sour pickles or sugary pastries. Many of the large companies that make processed foods are concerned with consumer's needs, wishes, and buying practices. Decaffeinated coffee, for example, arose because of consumer concern over the effects of caffeine. Margarine has largely replaced butter in many households because of concern over the health effects of saturated fat. Few people today cook or bake with lard. It has been almost entirely replaced by vegetable oil shortenings, corn oil and safflower oil, which are also used in frying and for salad dressings. Even highly processed foods are being put out in altered or modified forms, such as "imitation" mayonnaise, which is much lower in cholesterol than ordinary mayonnaise. Furthermore, many of these products are easily obtained in any supermarket.

Therefore, the problem confronting a young woman who uses processed foods in a dietary program for fitness, weight maintenance or weight loss is to find those foods that are convenient while still satisfying the basic rules of the program—foods low in calories, low in fat, low in refined sugar and with a high nutrient density. The label is the key to the nutrient density of the food. How much vitamin B or vitamin C or iron is there per calorie? As examples, let us take two processed foods. Brand X contains 150 calories per serving and 15 percent of the daily requirement for vitamins A and C and iron. Brand Y contains 75 calories per serving and 10 percent of the daily requirements for the same vitamins. On the basis of nutrient density—vitamins and iron per calorie—brand Y wins, it will give her 20 percent rather than 15 percent of her vitamin requirements per 150 calories; thus, even though a serving of brand X provides more of the vitamins in question than a serving of brand Y, the latter is the better product for a young woman concerned with meeting her nutrient needs while keeping her calories at a minimum.

However, the overall nutrient density of a processed food, while important, may in many cases not be as important as the specific nutrients the food contains. In the case of most nutrients, for example, there is no reason to consume more than 100 percent of the daily requirement. Therefore, if a particular nutrient is so widely available in foods that deficiencies of it rarely if ever occur, its density in a processed food is much less important than is the density of a nutrient that is in short supply in the diet. As we have seen, iron, folic acid, calcium and zinc are four nutrients that tend to be in short supply in the diets of many young women, and their density in processed foods should be given particular attention when reading labels.

Perhaps more important than any nutrients that may be missing from a processed food is the quantity and type of the nutrients that it contains. Many processed foods have high fat contents and contain large amounts of refined sugar for sweetening, whereas, as we have seen, both fat and refined sugar should be reduced in a diet emphasizing weight control and fitness. Furthermore there is evidence, as has already been mentioned and which we will examine in greater detail in Chapter 7, that too much fat in the diet is associated with heart disease and breast cancer, while excessive salt consumption has been associated with high blood pressure (hypertension), another major killer. Yet excess fat and excess salt are two problems with many processed foods. Canned peas, for instance, may seem much more convenient than fresh peas or even frozen peas, but they also may contain one hundred times more salt. Cold cuts are also very convenient, but such meats as bacon, salami, pastrami and the like are extremely high in both fat and salt. Pickled foods and smoked foods are loaded with salt.

Since none of the foregoing diseases is frequent in young women, with whom this chapter is concerned, you may wonder why I raise this subject here. My reason is that these diseases take many years to develop, and to the extent that excessive salt or fat contributes to their development, the earlier such excess is eliminated the better.

Fortunately, people have begun to ask questions about the nutrient content of food, to read labels and most important to buy food with its nutritional content in mind. The major food processors are therefore becoming more and more concerned about nutrition because it is good business. Fortunately, too, young women are their most important customers, since they will be buying for a long time, and if they buy those products that are nutritionally most sound for themselves and their families, and cut down on those that are not, the companies will get the message and will probably respond.

I am not naive enough to believe that food will be chosen solely for its nutritional value. Nor am I sure that this would always be appropriate. I am not even suggesting that foods always be chosen primarily for their nutritional value. But certainly other things being equal, a young woman can choose the product or the brand that makes the most nutritional sense. It may take a little time to read those labels but from the standpoint of health, it is time well spent.

DINING OUT

More than 20 percent of the meals Americans eat are consumed outside the home. This figure is considerably higher among young adults, particularly before they have any children. Therefore, if you are engaged in a dietary program for fitness it is important that what you eat in restaurants be part of that program. Dining out can be fun. It also can offer good nutrition. But certain simple rules are worth remembering: cocktails and wine provide calories that must be counted as part of the overall caloric content of the meal; the meal should include some high-nutrient-density foods, such as salads or certain fruits and vegetables; whole grains in the form of bread, rice and pastas will deliver many nutrients per calorie; avoid fatty cuts of meat and deep-fried foods; creamed soups, sauces and rich desserts are usually high in fat and therefore of low nutrient density.

Luckily, the wide choices of food available at most restaurants permit eating a combination of foods that satisfies even the most discriminating palate while at the same time conforming to a dietary program for fitness, even in restaurants that serve foods quite different from those that we may generally be used to. Furthermore, when compared to the usual fast-food restaurant, the choices in such restaurants are wider and the food generally contains less fat and fewer calories, and often is of a higher nutrient density. Italian, Chinese, Middle Eastern, Greek, Mexican, Spanish, Japanese and Indian foods, for example, offer a wide array of tastes and combinations, and can also offer excellent nutrition if the right choices are made. Pasta, the mainstay of many Italian meals, is essentially complex carbohydrate, but if made from enriched flour also contains abundant amounts of B vitamins. A salad with Italian dressing is rich in folic acid and vitamin C, and the meat dishes in an Italian restaurant, particularly veal, are low in fat and high in iron, zinc and vitamin B_{12}. Watch the bread, butter and desserts, however; Italian desserts are often high in fat and in calories.

Chinese food offers such variety that dishes can be found to suit practically every palate and dietary pattern. Unfortunately, one problem with Chinese food (and also Japanese food) is that it is high in sodium, which can be a problem for people with a tendency to high blood pressure. Mexican food features many meat, grain (often corn) and bean specialties, a great number of which are of high nutrient density. In fact, in literally every type of ethnic restaurant, dishes can be found that fit the active lifestyle of today's young woman. And eating in such restaurants, especially when combined with meeting people of different backgrounds, can be a new and pleasing experience.

ALTERNATIVE DIETS

In their quest for fitness, many young women experiment with many different kinds of diets. Some adopt alternative eating patterns with which they stay for long periods, in some cases throughout life. But while many of these diets are not only acceptable, but much more healthful than the average American diet, others are too restrictive and may result in nutrient deficiencies.

Vegetarianism Vegetarianism has become very popular among young people. Large segments of the student bodies at many universities, for example, are practicing vegetarians, and the custom is spreading rapidly. There is no reason for concern with this, since even the strictest vegetarian diet can supply excellent nutrition, and a young woman who decides to try this eating pattern can select a diet that will be both satisfying and healthful. First, however, it is important for her to learn something about vegetarianism so that she can be sure her diet supplies her with the nutrients needed for fitness and health.

There are two types of vegetarians: those who eat only foods derived from plants (vegans), and those who eat no meat but who will eat milk products. Vegetarians of the latter type who eat milk and milk products are called lacto-vegetarians; those who eat only eggs and plant-derived foods are called ovo-vegetarians; and those who eat eggs, milk and milk products are called ovo-lacto-vegetarians. If adequate amounts of eggs, milk and cheese are eaten, they will provide large enough amounts of protein, iron, calcium and vitamin B_{12} to meet all of the requirements for these nutrients, which exist only in potentially low amounts in plants. Such a diet will also be high in calcium and low in phosphorus, and will therefore favor calcium absorption. The only danger with such a diet is that, depending on the quantity of dairy foods eaten, it may be high in saturated fat. If this is the case, simply using skimmed milk, limiting the number of egg yolks and substituting margarine for butter should solve the problem. Therefore, no special precautions need be taken by a young woman who is an ovo-lacto-vegetarian. This is not only a healthful way to eat, but probably much more healthful than the average American diet. On the other hand, certain problems can be anticipated—and avoided with proper precautions—in a young woman who decides to become a vegan or a strict vegetarian, excluding all meat, poultry, fish, milk and their products from her diet. The major difficulty with a strict vegetarian diet is that protein from plant sources is usually incomplete, versus the completeness of most animal proteins, which contain all of the eight essential amino acids that the body cannot manufacture. An exception to this is the protein found in soybeans, which—in terms of the essential amino acids—is as good as some animal-derived protein.

Moreover, those essential amino acids that are present only in small amounts or are missing in plants such as grains are abundant in other plants such as legumes. One can therefore obtain all of the essential amino acids in a single meal simply by combining different plant foods containing various proteins. This practice is called "complementing proteins." For example, grains, which generally have a low content of the amino acid lysine and a high content of the amino acid methionine, can be combined with legumes, which have a low methionine but a high lysine content.

The concept of complementing proteins is not new. In fact, it is probably through this practice that most civilizations that ate very little meat were able to survive. It is no accident, for example, that Latin Americans regularly eat meals containing both corn tortillas (a grain) and red beans (a legume). Other plant-protein-derived amino acids can be combined in a like manner to form complete proteins. Of course the addition of even small amounts of protein from animal sources to a meal increases its total protein value. Figure 1 is a general guide to follow when complementing proteins.

One nutrient that is available only from animal sources

FIGURE 2

FOODS
THAT
COMPLEMENT
PROTEINS

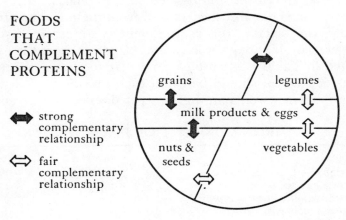

→ strong
complementary
relationship

⇔ fair
complementary
relationship

From: Nutrition and Health, *ed. M. Winick, Vol. 2, No. 1, 1980.*

is vitamin B_{12}, which is important for producing new red blood cells. Thus, a strict vegetarian will become deficient in this vitamin. Furthermore, since the symptoms of this deficiency can take a long time (up to several years) to develop, the deficiency itself and the serious anemia that accompanies it can easily be overlooked until its late stages. Because of this, it is extremely important that any young woman consuming a vegan diet be provided with a source of vitamin B_{12}. Brewer's yeast, tempeh (a fermented soybean product) and fortified breakfast cereals are all good sources, and usually acceptable to vegetarians. If these foods are not eaten regularly, a vitamin B_{12} supplement should be used.

As discussed earlier, women during their reproductive years are at risk for iron deficiency, and this risk is increased if they are on a vegetarian diet. Therefore, certain plant foods that contain significant amounts of iron (see

Table 4) should be emphasized in a vegetarian diet. But since iron is not absorbed as well from these foods as from meat, the dietary iron requirement is higher in a strict vegetarian. If enough iron cannot be gotten from the foods listed in Table 4 because of particular food preferences, a fortified cereal should be eaten each morning or an iron supplement (twenty milligrams per day) should be taken.

TABLE 4   IRON CONTENT OF PLANT FOODS

FOOD	AMOUNT	IRON (MG)
Enriched white rice (cooked)	1 cup	1.8
Brown rice (cooked)	1 cup	1.0
Bread (whole wheat and white)	1 slice	0.7
Spinach (cooked)	1 cup	4.8
Kale (cooked)	1 cup	1.3
Tofu (soybean curd)	1 piece	2.3
Beans (e.g., kidney)	1 cup	4.5
Peanut butter	2 tbsp.	0.6
Bean sprouts (raw)	1 cup	1.4
Brewer's yeast	1 tbsp.	1.4
Torula yeast	1 oz.	5.5
Fruit (e.g., banana)	1	1.0
Dried fruit (e.g., raisins)	1½ oz.	1.5

The same general rules hold for calcium as for iron. Women of college age are still building their calcium reserves and therefore require large amounts of this nutrient in their diets. Calcium is supplied mainly by dairy products (see Figure 2), and if no dairy products are being consumed within a vegetarian diet, particular attention must be paid to the plant sources of calcium shown in Table 5. Alternatively, a calcium supplement can be taken. Five hundred milligrams of calcium, usually in the form of a calcium gluconate tablet, is adequate for this purpose.

From the foregoing discussion, it can be seen that a young woman, whether a vegan or an ovo-lacto vegetarian, can consume a healthful and varied diet with only minor

FIGURE 2

CALCIUM SOURCES

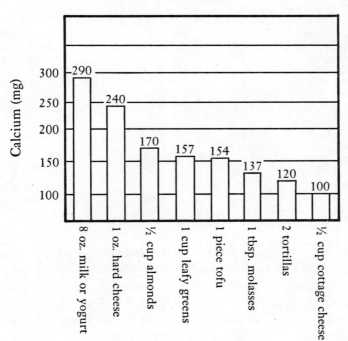

From: Nutrition and Health, *ed. M. Winick, Vol. 2, No. 1, 1980.*

TABLE 5   **FOODS HIGH IN CALCIUM**
(Each Portion Provides About 300 mg of Calcium)

FOOD	SERVING SIZE
Almonds, chopped	1 cup
Amaranth	4 oz.
Broccoli	2¼ cups
Cheese	
Cottage	12 oz.
Cheddar	1½ oz.
Sandwich type	2 oz.

FOOD	SERVING SIZE
Collard greens, chopped, cooked	1 cup
Custard	1 cup
Fish (canned)*	
Mackerel	3½ oz.
Salmon	5½ oz.
Sardines	3½ oz.
Ice cream	1⅔ cup
Kale	2 cups
Kelp	1½ oz.
Milk	
Whole, low-fat or buttermilk	8 oz.
Evaporated	4 oz.
Tofu (soybean curd)	8 oz.
Tortillas (6 in. diameter)	5
Turnip greens	1½ cups
Yeast (brewers)	14 tbsp.
Yogurt	¾ cup

*Includes the softened bones

adjustments. Such diets have the advantage of being high in their fiber content and, in the case of vegetarians consuming only occasional dairy products, relatively low in calories and in total and saturated fat. And since these are dietary goals that all of us should be striving for, there is no reason to discourage vegetarianism.

A variation of the vegetarian diet—quite common on college campuses and gaining in popularity among the population in general—is the diet that excludes meat but permits fowl, fish, seafood and dairy products. Such a diet has plenty of protein, is relatively low in fat, and is high in complex carbohydrate and in dietary fiber. It is a very healthful diet that approaches the dietary guidelines set for Americans by the Departments of Health and Human Services and of Agriculture. This diet not only offers more variety than a vegetarian diet, but will much more easily supply the requirements for iron, zinc and vitamin B_{12}. Moreover, the animal protein in the diet permits the body to use the vegetable protein without the extensive complementing that must be done on a strict vegetarian diet. Finally, this type of diet is generally low in calories, primarily because it is low in fat and high in bulk. It therefore fits into an active lifestyle, including snacking, dining out, and using processed foods. For the young woman concerned with her weight, it is therefore an excellent diet. In fact, it is one possible choice in the dietary pattern for fitness outlined earlier in this chapter.

RESTRICTIVE DIETS

Some young people, as part of their search for change, their feeling of the need to reject established patterns, and their desire to experiment with new things, adopt dietary regimens that can be dangerous. High on the list of these is the so-called Zen Macrobiotic diet. This diet progresses through stages from a simple vegetarian regimen that allows some animal products to one consisting entirely of rice and herb tea. The more restrictive phases, if maintained for any length of time, can be extremely dangerous. The diet is deficient in protein, vitamin D, iron, calcium and vitamin C, among other nutrients, and cases of protein-calorie malnutrition with stunted growth, rickets, scurvy and severe anemia have all been reported in persons following this diet. There are many ways to experiment with new patterns of living without endangering your health, and the Zen Macrobiotic diet is not one of them. Therefore, if you know someone planning to undertake such a diet, try to discourage her.

Another commonly practiced diet involves eating only those foods that have been grown "organically." The definition of an organic food is not always clear. Most often what is meant is that no artificial fertilizer has been used and no pesticides employed in its growth. Certainly there is nothing wrong with consuming such foods, but no health advantages have been documented for them, and they are far more expensive than foods grown in the ordinary manner. Furthermore, depending on the health of the supplying animal, the use of so-called organic fertilizers such as manure can carry certain dangers. And while the absence of pesticides is desirable it is doubtful, within our highly mechanized agricultural society, that without some form of insect control as well as "artificial" fertilizer we could grow sufficient food to supply the world's needs. The recent fruit fly infestation of a large part of California's growing belt, which threatened to wreak havoc on the entire economy of that state and affect the food supply of the entire country, and for which the only solution proved to be the use of pesticides, is proof of this. Therefore, rather than avoiding the use of pesticides and artificial fertilizer entirely, what must be done is to establish strict controls on these materials and an efficient and effective system for monitoring their safety. The use of organically grown foods may be a solution for the relatively rich who can afford to eat that way, but for the hundreds of millions of people throughout the world whose only chance for a decent life depends on increased agricultural productivity, this is certainly no answer.

For a young woman, the period of transition from adolescence to adulthood ends when a new home and family are established. Most often this means marriage (although growing numbers of couples are living together without marrying), and the beginning of a new lifestyle. No longer is the young woman concerned only with her own life; she must now also be concerned with that of her husband. A new chapter in her life has begun.

ORAL CONTRACEPTIVES AND NUTRITION

Sometime before or during the period of marriage and the beginning of a family, a young woman must make a very personal decision. Does she wish to practice contraception, and if so, what method does she wish to use? Many women, for a variety of reasons, elect to use contraceptive pills until they and their husbands decide to have children.

Oral contraceptives are hormones, usually a combination of estrogen and progesterone, that block the normal female hormonal cycle and thereby prevent ovulation. In most cases they also reduce the amount of bleeding associated with menstruation. Since hormones are very potent substances with wide effects on the metabolism of the body, any young woman who decides to use oral contraceptives should consult her physician, who can help her choose the preparation that is best for her. More important, from the viewpoint of our discussion here, is that any woman planning to use these preparations should be aware of the nutritional dangers they can present and of what can be done to avoid them.

The use of oral contraceptives has produced a number of nutritional problems in at least some women of childbearing age. Because these preparations reduce the blood loss in menstruation, the loss of iron will also be lower and the dietary iron requirement will decrease. Additionally, there is evidence that vitamin A levels in the blood increase in many women taking oral contraceptives, suggesting that such women also have a lower dietary vitamin A requirement. On the other side of the coin, women taking contraceptive pills often have lower folic acid levels in their blood, which can be very dangerous for a woman whose diet is already deficient in folic acid and who continues to consume such a diet. Anemia caused by folic acid deficiency can and does occur in such cases.

Another vitamin that can become deficient in women who use oral contraceptives is pyridoxine (vitamin B_6), and a frank deficiency of this nutrient can occur if its concentration in the blood is low prior to starting on the pill. Other vitamins whose concentrations have been shown to be lower than normal in many women using oral contraceptives—but to a much smaller degree than folic acid and vitamin B_6—are thiamine, riboflavin and vitamin B_{12}. Because folic acid and vitamin B_6 deficiency can be serious matters, we shall concern ourselves primarily with these two vitamins.

Foods rich in folic acid are lacking in the diets of many young women (see Table 6), who for this reason tend to have low levels of this important nutrient, especially if they are taking oral contraceptives. Any woman who has been on oral contraceptives for any length of time should therefore be checked for anemia once a year, and should begin immediate treatment with folic acid tablets if she is found to be anemic as a result of folic acid deficiency. One dietary solution to preventing such deficiency is the use of fortified cereals containing folic acid. Many do not. With regard to this, a cereal that has 25 percent or more of the RDA of folic acid should be chosen, as revealed by the label. The cereal should be one that has not been fortified with vitamin A (or one that has more than 15 percent of the RDA for vitamin A), but should be fortified with pyridoxine (which is the case for most cereals). Another solution is to take a vitamin pill containing both folic acid and pyridoxine in small doses. The problem with such pills is that most also contain vitamin A. Finally, an emphasis can be put on foods generally containing folic acid.

The problem with vitamin B_6 is less urgent than that

TABLE 6	FOLIC ACID CONTENT OF FOODS IN MICROGRAMS (mcg) PER SERVING				

5–20 MCG/SERVING			20–50 MCG/SERVING	
carrot	1 med.		green beans	1 cup
ear of corn	1 med.		cucumber	1 small
mushrooms	3 large		squash	⅔ cup
potato	1 med.		strawberries	1 cup
apple	1 med.		egg	1 large
hard cheese	1 oz.		kidney	3 oz.
grapefruit	½ med.		shell fish	6 oz.
milk	8 oz.		yogurt	8 oz.
bread	1 slice			
sesame seeds	1 tbsp.			
lean beef, veal or pork	6 oz.			

100–150 MCG/SERVING			200–300 MCG/SERVING	
liver (all)	3 oz.		brewer's yeast	1 tbsp.
broccoli	2 stalks		spinach	4 oz.
orange juice	6 oz.			

From: Nutrition and Health, *ed. M. Winick, Vol. 4, No. 1, 1982.*

with folic acid because deficiency of this vitamin in the general population is less common. However, since various nonspecific symptoms, such as feelings of depression, have in many cases been traced to vitamin B_6 deficiency, any woman exhibiting such symptoms should have her vitamin B_6 status checked. During pregnancy, both folic acid and vitamin B_6 are particularly important for adequate growth and development of the fetus, and any woman who becomes pregnant shortly after stopping the use of contraceptive pills should therefore receive supplements of these two vitamins throughout her pregnancy.

Another frequent complaint of women taking oral contraceptives is weight gain. This is usually due to the accumulation of water, not fat, and hence cannot be controlled by dietary means. Women in whom such a problem becomes severe should seek the advice of their doctor, who may prescribe a different oral contraceptive preparation to eliminate the problem.

A final nutritional concern for women taking contraceptive pills is the effect that alcohol and certain drugs can have in combination with these hormonal preparations. Alcohol can reduce the absorption of both folic acid and vitamin B_6, and a woman who is a heavy alcohol user and is also taking the pill must therefore take supplements of these vitamins. Most notable among the drugs that can affect folic acid metabolism is dilantin, an antiepileptic drug. No woman who takes this drug should take an oral contraceptive other than under a doctor's care. The same is true for women taking isoniazid, a common antituberculosis drug, since this drug can cause vitamin B_6 deficiency and markedly accentuate any B_6 deficiency caused by an oral contraceptive.

PREPARING FOR GROWTH OF THE FAMILY

So far, I have spoken positively of the new and active lifestyle that begins after adolescence and continues with the newly married couple. Nevertheless, there are several troublesome aspects of this lifestyle, particularly among young women. One of these is the smoking habit.

Save for young women, among whom cigarette smoking continues to increase, smoking has declined among all segments of the general population. Beyond the obvious health hazards associated with this habit—including cancer of the lung, emphysema (damaged air sacs in the lungs) and coronary heart disease—cigarette smoking affects the nutritional status of a young woman. For example, there is evidence that vitamin C levels are lower in the blood of cigarette smokers than nonsmokers, suggesting that smoking depletes this vitamin. Furthermore, smoking is particularly dangerous during pregnancy, when, even if only moderate, it will adversely affect the nutrition of the fetus. And since it is very difficult for a woman to stop smoking once she is pregnant, if you smoke and are planning to have a baby, the time to quit is now.

Smoking marijuana is another habit that may begin in adolescence and continue through the early days of independence. Like cigarette smoking, this habit is also potentially dangerous during pregnancy, and should also be broken before conception.

Going beyond marijuana, some young women have experimented with hard drugs during adolescence or in young adulthood, and some may continue to "experiment" with these substances into marriage. Drug use at any time is a serious problem requiring medical help. However, it is particularly serious during pregnancy. Infants born to addicted mothers often show severe withdrawal symptoms after birth, and some die. Therefore, if you take hard drugs, get help, and do not get pregnant until you have completely conquered the habit.

The problem of alcoholism is another major public health concern in America, exposing the many young women who drink heavily to both the direct toxic effects of alcohol and the risk of severe nutritional difficulties. I am not talking about the occasional drink or glass of wine with dinner, but rather the two or three cocktails before dinner, the after dinner drink or two, the nightcap and the many variations of this theme.

We have already noted that alcohol is a significant source of empty calories, and that its consumption therefore interferes with the ability to obtain required nutrients. Beyond this, however, alcohol interferes with the absorption and metabolism of specific nutrients—often the very ones that are in shortest supply in a young woman's diet. It will impair the absorption of folic acid, and heavy drinkers often develop the anemia that follows folic acid deficiency.

A young woman whose diet is marginal for this vitamin to begin with is therefore especially at risk for folic acid deficiency if she drinks moderately—let alone heavily—and is in even greater danger if she is taking contraceptive pills.

Thiamine (vitamin B_1) deficiency has almost completely disappeared in America except among people who are heavy drinkers, in whom heart failure and brain damage caused by deficiency in this vitamin are very serious problems. Similarly, the metabolism of pyridoxine (vitamin B_6) is also adversely affected by alcohol. Again this vitamin is particularly important in women during the reproductive years.

Two further nutrients in which alcohol can induce a deficiency are iron and zinc—both of which—like folic acid and the B vitamins—are critical during pregnancy. One effect of chronic alcohol use is an often unnoticeable microscopic bleeding from the gastrointestinal tract which, over a long period of time, will result in iron depletion and iron deficiency anemia. Alcohol consumption also reduces the amount of zinc absorbed from foods, thereby inducing zinc deficiency. For such reasons, it is clearly obvious that heavy drinking is not only particularly dangerous in young women of childbearing age, but incompatible with any program designed to keep a young woman fit.

There is some evidence that heavy coffee consumption during pregnancy may adversely affect fetal growth. Certainly three or four cups are safe, but if you are a ten cup a day coffee drinker, begin to cut back before you become pregnant.

Two further nutritional matters are of concern to the young woman planning to become pregnant: She should be as close to her ideal weight as possible before becoming pregnant, and—for the reasons discussed earlier—if she has been taking contraceptive pills for any length of time she should spend some time replenishing her supply of certain nutrients before coming off the pill, and should continue this supplementation into and during her pregnancy.

We will discuss the importance of adequate weight gain during pregnancy in the next chapter. Here, however, it is worth noting that many young women, concerned about their weight, have dropped to a level below what is ideal for them, and sometimes considerably below this. If you are among these women, you would be wise to gain a little weight before becoming pregnant. It will reduce the number of pounds you will have to gain during pregnancy in order to be able to nourish your fetus well. The table on 174 is an ideal weight table for women of various heights who are of childbearing age. Find your ideal weight and try to approach it before becoming pregnant.

The woman who is overweight should lose weight before becoming pregnant. While an overweight woman needs to gain somewhat less weight during her pregnancy, she must still gain a significant amount, and may therefore end her pregnancy at an undesirably high weight, if she enters pregnancy significantly overweight to begin with. The next chapter is about pregnancy itself, a period unique to a woman's life, and one that has very special nutritional requirements.

CHAPTER 5

When You Are Pregnant

*T*he time has come. You and your husband have decided to have a child. Ideally you will enter pregnancy in the best possible condition both psychologically and physically. You will be close to or at your ideal weight and will have achieved this before becoming pregnant. If you have been using contraceptive pills you will have begun taking a vitamin supplement before stopping your use of them. Henceforth your drinking should be limited, your smoking brought down to a minimum and your use of drugs of any kind stopped altogether. From now on nature will largely take care of the rest.

The continuum of pregnancy and lactation has evolved over millions of years. They are not "special conditions" requiring extreme care. If left to its own devices, any mammal with an abundance of food will almost always deliver a healthy offspring and be able to nurse it until it is capable of an independent existence, and biologically, you are no exception to this. Your body has learned over the millennia to become a finely tuned instrument that senses immediately when you are pregnant and responds quickly by beginning a process of adaptation that will provide just the right environment for your developing fetus.

ADAPTING TO PREGNANCY

Expanding your blood supply Unlike the egg of a bird, which contains ample food for the growth of its embryo into a chick, the fertilized mammalian egg carries only enough reserve food to nourish a growing embryo for a few days. Thus, while the bird can simply sit on her eggs and provide them with warmth, you must provide your developing embryo with food and oxygen carried by your blood, and must rid its growing body of the waste products that it produces. The complex machinery necessary for this two-way transfer system is set up during the earliest stage of pregnancy. While the fertilized ovum is still passing from the ovary to its home in the uterus, the wall of the latter organ prepares to accept its tiny occupant. The uterine blood vessels begin to enlarge, supplying more blood to the uterine tissues and cells. Initially this is accomplished by a redistribution of blood from some of the other organs of the body. But because the uterus and the embryo within it are growing at a very rapid rate, the total volume of blood circulating through your body must also increase rapidly in order to accommodate that growth. Thus, one of the first adaptations that your body makes in pregnancy is to increase its blood volume.

The increase in the body's blood volume in early pregnancy is not a sudden accumulation of new blood, but a gradual adding to the blood that is already circulating in the body. The increase begins early and continues well into pregnancy. By the time you have fully adapted, in about the eighth month, your blood volume will have increased by 50 percent, or more than two extra pints of blood. Most of this new blood will be directed first to the reproductive organs and later to the enlarging breasts. Your body also responds to its newly increased blood volume in a unique manner. Your heart begins to pump more blood with each contraction, so that even though there is more blood to circulate, the rate at which it moves through your body is kept the same. This increase in what is called the "cardiac output" ensures that nutrients and oxygen are delivered to the tissues at a proper rate. Bathed by this nutrient-rich blood, which is also supplied in greater amounts, your uterus begins to enlarge, and its cells form the bed on which your embryo will grow and develop into a fetus during the next nine months (ten lunar months).

The placenta The placenta is the only organ in the animal kingdom that grows from two distinct individuals; it develops in all mammals when they become pregnant. Part of it originates from the mother's uterine tissues and part from a specialized portion of the embryo. In many ways this extremely specialized organ with its very limited lifespan and specific mission is the most remarkable organ in the mammalian kingdom. For example, its two parts (maternal and fetal), while in intimate contact, remain separate so that the blood from the mother and that of the fetus—both of which circulate through the placenta—never mix. The placenta also carries out many essential metabolic reactions; it produces hormones, transfers nutrients and oxygen from the mother's blood supply to that of the fetus, and moves carbon dioxide and waste products from the blood of the fetus to that of the mother. It therefore keeps the developing fetus constantly supplied with its needs and maintains the conditions that ensure its best possible growth and development. Yet although the placenta has fascinated scientists for centuries, only recently have many of its most important functions been understood.

A two-way street Perhaps the most important job of the placenta is to transfer substances to and from the fetus. In this role it functions as a combined intestine, lung and kidney, constantly transferring nutrients and oxygen from the increased maternal circulation to the developing fetal circulation, while passing carbon dioxide and other waste products from the fetal blood to the mother's blood, from which they are then eliminated through the mother's lungs and kidneys. Some substances, such as oxygen and carbon dioxide, simply pass directly through the thin membrane in the placenta that separates the mother's circulation from that of her infant. Other substances, such as simple sugars and amino acids (the building blocks of protein), must be helped across by a process called active transport. These substances attach themselves to specialized molecules made by the placenta, and known as "carrier molecules," which then carry them across the thin placental membrane, releasing them on the other side. Some nutrients may share the same carrier molecule; others have carrier molecules that are constructed to fit them uniquely.

If the active transport system of the placenta is thought of as a continuous railroad that picks up its cargo on the mother's side and discharges it on the baby's side (and vice versa in the case of waste products) it can be seen that the railroad must be powered by fuel or energy. Much of this fuel is created in the placenta from nutrients extracted from the mother's blood. Obviously, then, in order to have a well-nourished fetus you must first have a well-functioning and well-nourished placenta.

At this point you may ask why such a complicated arrangement is necessary for the development of your fetus. Why don't the two blood supplies simply mix, and the fetus extract what it needs? The answer to this is perhaps best explained by examining another important function of the placenta.

The great protector No two babies, with the exception of identical twins, are genetically alike. Your fetus contains genes that come from both you and your husband; they direct and regulate the development of its tissues and organs, and ensure that these tissues and organs are different from those of either parent. It is in this way that nature assures maximum diversity within any species. The components of the fetus's blood are also unique, and the specialized immune system that protects it against disease, when formed, will recognize unfamiliar substances—including some of those that are part of its mother's cells and tissues —as "foreign," and will mobilize defenses to expel these invading entities.

The protective function of the placenta can best be understood by using the example of a blood transfusion. Because of its genetic makeup, your fetus may have a different type of blood from yours, and if the two blood supplies were mixed, either you or the fetus could have a severe reaction, as sometimes happens when the wrong type of blood is given in a transfusion. Occasionally this happens when a small number of fetal blood cells "leak" across the placental barrier into the blood of a mother who has a different blood type. If even this small "transfusion" can cause problems for the fetus, even greater mixing of the two blood supplies could cause the death of many fetuses and seriously affect many mothers as well. But to prevent such potentially serious reaction is not the only function of the "placental barrier"; it also keeps out infectious bacteria, viruses and agents within the mother's blood that might be noxious to the fetus.

Finally, if the placenta did not keep the maternal and fetal blood supplies separate, the mother and the fetus would be competing for the same nutrients. And because the requirements of the fetus for many nutrients are much higher than at any other time of life, every fetal organ would have to be able to extract these nutrients from the mother's blood more rapidly than they could be extracted by the mother's own tissues. Instead, the placenta does the whole job, partitioning the nutrients not according to their availability alone, but also according to the needs of both the mother and the fetus. If the fetus's need for vitamin C, for example, is greater than the mother's, the placenta carries extra vitamin C to the fetus and the fetal blood becomes richer in vitamin C than the maternal blood.

I hope you are beginning to get a sense of the truly astounding nature of the placenta. But even this is only part of the story.

The master gland of pregnancy While the hormones produced by your pituitary gland and ovaries initiate pregnancy, it is largely the hormones produced by the placenta that maintain pregnancy. These placental hormones affect your body in a variety of ways: They help maintain the proper conditions for your fetus to thrive; they help stimulate the development of your breast tissues so that you will be able to nurse your infant when he or she is born; and there is some evidence that the placenta in some way senses when the fetus is ready to be born and releases hormones that trigger the beginning of labor.

Some of the hormones produced by the placenta are for fetal use. For example, before the fetal adrenal gland can function properly, the placenta manufactures certain "adrenal" (cortisone-like) hormones that the fetus needs. The placenta also produces its own growth hormone (placental lactogen), which helps regulate the growth of the young fetus. And in at least one instance the placenta goes into partnership with the fetus to produce a vital hormone. One important hormone that is a derivative of cortisone and is normally made in the adult adrenal cortex is only partially made in the fetal adrenal cortex. The incomplete and inactive fetal hormone is secreted into the fetal blood stream, from which it goes to the placenta where specialized tissue completes the job. The complete and now functional hormone is then passed back into the fetal bloodstream, which carries it to all of the fetal tissues.

Lastly, pregnancy is a time when both the mother and the fetus need calcium, and there is a hormone that regulates calcium metabolism and helps calcium to be properly deposited in bone, and which is normally made only in the kidney, from vitamin D obtained either in the diet or from the skin. (We will discuss this hormone in greater detail later in this chapter, and again when we examine the brittle bone condition known as osteoporosis that is common in older women.) Recent evidence suggests that even though the mother's kidneys produce this hormone actively, the placenta also produces the hormone, increasing its concentration in the mother's blood and thereby permitting efficient regulation of both her own calcium metabolism and bone structure and that of her fetus at a time when calcium is particularly important.

The placenta, then, is a hormone factory, manufacturing its own hormones for both the mother and the fetus, augmenting the supply of hormones made by the mother, and helping the fetus complete the synthesis of certain vital hormones that it cannot yet synthesize by itself.

Because the placenta is the vital lifeline between you and your baby during almost the entire course of pregnancy, and because in early pregnancy it grows more rapidly than the fetus, poor placental growth will almost inevitably lead to poor fetal growth. Some other adaptations that your body makes during pregnancy are therefore important in ensuring proper growth of both the placenta and the fetus.

Bringing in the nutrients One of the most important adaptations that your body makes during pregnancy—one that is important for the nutrition of both you and your fetus—takes place within your gastrointestinal tract. The rate at which the gastrointestinal tract absorbs iron and calcium from the foods you consume limits the rate at which these two important nutrients enter your body. Normally about 10 percent of the iron and 20 to 30 percent of the calcium in your diet is absorbed. During pregnancy, however, the absorption of these nutrients is markedly increased because they are so important to both the mother and the fetus. We still do not understand the mechanism by which this increase occurs in the case of iron, and our information with regard to calcium is very limited. But what we do know is fascinating and illustrates how the mother's kidneys, in partnership with the placenta, influence her gastrointestinal tract to absorb more calcium, and how the increased need of both the mother and the fetus for calcium triggers the entire process.

As mentioned briefly in the previous section, calcium metabolism is regulated by a hormone made from vitamin D, which is converted in two steps (first in the liver and then in the kidney) to an active hormone. The kidney then releases this hormone into the bloodstream, in which it travels to the gastrointestinal (G.I.) tract and the bones, where it exerts its activity. In the gastrointestinal tract, where most of its activity occurs, the vitamin D hormone (dihydroxycholecalciferol) promotes the absorption of calcium from the food into the blood. It does this by influencing the cells that line the gastrointestinal tract to make a protein that is thought to help carry the calcium through the walls of the tract and release it into the blood. In bone, where the hormone is also active, it helps in the process of calcification, which creates the hardness necessary for the bones to support the weight of the body.

The concentration of calcium in the blood controls how much of the hormone the kidney makes. When the calcium levels in the blood are low, the kidney makes more hormone, prompting more calcium to be taken into the body. This calcium then reaches the bones, where some of it is deposited. When calcium is not coming in from the outside, the large supply of calcium in the bones, besides serving as a structural component, also serves as a vast "reservoir" that supplies the blood with this mineral. Thus, to keep its level of calcium high and the rest of the tissues supplied, the blood can take in calcium from two sources—the food in the gastrointestinal tract and the bones. The source it uses depends on the amount of dihydroxycholecalciferol made in the kidney, which in turn depends on the amount of calcium in the blood.

During pregnancy, not only does the kidney make more of the vitamin D hormone, but—as we have already noted —the placenta also makes the hormone. How and why this occurs is not understood, but as a consequence, the level of the hormone in the maternal blood will be very high. The mother's calcium absorption will therefore increase, and more calcium will be available to the rapidly forming fetal skeleton. Normally this process is so efficient that there is not only enough calcium available for your fetus but enough left over to strengthen your own bones.

If you consume insufficient amounts of vitamin D and if you do not get enough sunlight to activate the vitamin in your skin, the amount of dihydroxycholecalciferol produced in both the kidney and the placenta will be reduced. However, excess dietary vitamin D will not be converted to the hormone and can be toxic to you and to your fetus. Therefore, do not try to help nature by consuming large quantities of vitamin D. It won't work and it can be dangerous. On the other hand, the amount of calcium in the diet is important, and since calcium intake in many women is low, you may wish to increase the amount you consume.

Changes in other systems As your pregnancy proceeds, changes occur in your lungs and kidneys that increase the amount of oxygen you take in and the amount of carbon dioxide and waste products that you excrete. This increase satisfies the needs of the fetus and placenta. The amount of air you inhale and expire with each breath increases by about 30 percent. You actually breathe more deeply without any conscious effort to do so, and often without noticing it. Additionally, the kidney processes about 50 percent more blood per minute than it does before pregnancy, efficiently eliminating the waste products produced by the fetus and placenta. The increased output of urine that results from this, combined with the pressure on your bladder from the expanding uterus, explains the frequent need to urinate that occurs during pregnancy.

PREPARATION FOR NURSING

So far we have discussed only those adaptations that your body makes to nurture your developing fetus. However, it will also begin to make certain changes in preparation for nursing your infant after birth. It is important to remember that pregnancy and lactation are really a continuum—two parts of a single process—and that before the availability of infant formula the whole process had to proceed smoothly or the infant would not survive. Your body adapts in two ways to ensure that survival.

Breast development Under stimulation from the hormones that your body and placenta produce, your breasts begin to develop the capacity to produce milk. The blood supply to the glandular tissue within your breasts increases, and the veins on the surface of your breasts dilate to accommodate the increased blood supply. Your breast size increases and you may experience a sense of fullness or tenderness. From three-quarters of a pound to one and a half pounds of weight will have been added to each of your breasts by the time your pregnancy is over. Initially this weight increase is due to the weight of the extra blood. But by midpregnancy, the glands within the breast, which secrete the milk, also will have increased in size and number. Additionally, your breasts during the latter half of pregnancy will produce a thick liquid secretion called colostrum, which is extremely important to your infant in the early days after its birth, and which will add to the weight of your breasts and the feeling of heaviness as your term approaches. Toward the end of your pregnancy small amounts of colostrum may leak from your nipples. This is perfectly normal and is a sign that your breasts are ready for your hungry infant as soon as she or he arrives.

Fat deposition As we have already mentioned, fat will be deposited in your body during pregnancy. Do not be alarmed by this prospect; there is a very good reason for the deposition of this fat: It is an energy store for your infant when nursing begins. During pregnancy, between ten and fifteen pounds of fat will be deposited deep within your body. Since each pound of fat represents about 3,000 calories, you will have stored from thirty to forty-five thousand calories by the time you deliver your infant. And since your newborn infant will consume about five hundred calories per day, which will be supplied by your breast milk, you will have stored a two- to three-month supply of calories for your infant. This assumes that the conversion of your fat calories to your infant's milk calories is 100 percent efficient. However, it is not; energy must be expended (calories burned) in order to accomplish the fat-to-milk conversion, and the calories you have stored in the form of fat during your pregnancy will therefore be rapidly consumed during lactation.

If you are thinking "I'm not planning to breast feed so I don't need those calories and I'll limit my weight gain during pregnancy," don't! Nature doesn't know that you don't plan to nurse your infant. Evolution has not yet had time to deal with the phenomenon of bottle feeding. The

fat you require for milk production will be deposited any-
way, even at the expense of proper fetal growth, and you
certainly would not want that to happen.

Increasing your appetite Besides the energy-requiring adaptations that your own body makes to pregnancy, your fetus
and placenta are growing by constantly depositing new
tissue, your uterus has increased in size, your breasts have
enlarged and you have deposited about ten pounds of "lactation" fat—all of which also require energy and the building blocks necessary for new tissue growth. The energy is
supplied in the form of calories; the building blocks come
from dietary proteins and from some minerals; and vitamins and other minerals are necessary for tissues to grow.
In short, the requirements for all nutrients go up. Normally your body will sense this. After a short period in
which your food intake may go down and during which
many women complain of nausea, your appetite will increase.

The reason for this appetite increase remains a mystery,
but somehow all of the changes taking place in your body
signal the appetite control center in your brain, which in
turn sends a signal to your stomach and creates the feeling
of hunger. This increase in appetite is nature's way of
ensuring that fuel will be available for the complex adaptations that have evolved to provide your infant with a
healthy beginning. When we tamper with our desire to
consume more food, or when food is simply not available,
these adaptations will be incomplete and fetal growth may
be compromised. To guard against this it is important that
you eat the right amount and right kind of food.

Low birth weight Since nature has developed the complex
series of changes by which your body provides for the
adequate growth of your fetus, it is appropriate to ask why
it has gone to all that trouble. After all, suppose the fetus
is born a little smaller; it still has the rest of its life to catch

up. Why is the proper birth weight so important? The answer is that even with all our modern technology and our greater knowledge and understanding of the newborn, the best that medical science has to offer outside the uterus is still not nearly so good as what you have to offer inside it. Therefore, the better your infant grows in the womb the better its chances of surviving and of growing and developing properly after birth.

Let me illustrate how important adequate birth weight really is. The United States ranks fourteenth in infant mortality among the countries of the world; in thirteen other countries a newborn infant has a better chance of surviving than it does here. The reason for this relatively high mortality is the greater number of small babies that are born in the United States. Some persons might suggest that there are other factors; our population is racially more diverse than the Swedes, for example, and has many more poor people than in Denmark. On the surface this sounds logical; the single common denominator in the survival of American infants might appear to be socioeconomic status. But pound for pound the black baby does as well as the white baby, and the poor baby as well as the rich baby. The true difference is that the average birth weight in these poorer populations is one-half pound lighter than in the more affluent segments of our population. That one-half pound accounts entirely for our relatively high rate of infant mortality. Looking at it in another way, our overall infant mortality would approach that of the Scandinavian countries—which have the best record in the world—if we could raise the birth weight of our poorer populations by one-half pound, entirely eliminating the differences between rich and poor in this country.

Of course every infant, even under the best of circumstances, will not achieve the same birth weight; each has a certain potential for growth. Genetic factors in the infant and mother, for example, will influence the rate of fetal growth and therefore the birth weight. What we are trying to do is create the best conditions for your infant to achieve its potential. In order to do this it is important to understand those factors in your environment that are important influences on the growth of your fetus, for while there is little we can do about our genetic makeup, there is often much that can be done to improve our environment.

With regard to the growth of her fetus, the single most important factor in the mother's environment is her state of nutrition—both before and during pregnancy. From what we have seen earlier in this chapter, this should be no surprise. And yet the importance of maternal nutrition has only recently been fully understood.

MATERNAL NUTRITION

The importance of maternal nutrition to fetal health and survival was at least suspected as far back as the sixteenth century. Treatises of that time recognized that the fetus needed nutrients and that only the mother could supply them. At the same time, certain problems of overeating were also discussed. One complication often mentioned, which is interesting in view of future events, was the relation of "overeating" to large fetuses. In an early treatise on pregnancy the author cautions that overeating could cause "fetal outgrowth of the womb."

By the nineteenth and early twentieth century, the relationship of maternal diet to fetal growth was well known to physicians—so well known, in fact, that they attempted to influence fetal growth by restricting the mother's diet. At that time, the major concern during pregnancy was the mother's survival; maternal mortality was frighteningly high and methods of delivery were still primitive. Since larger babies were harder to deliver and so posed a greater risk to both the infant and the mother, it was felt that smaller babies were the solution, and that this could be achieved by restricting the amount of food the mother consumed. By the early and middle part of the twentieth century, obstetrics had improved markedly; maternal mortality almost entirely disappeared and deliveries became safer. But while the reason for limiting the mother's food intake thus disappeared, the practice remained. Rationales were created for continuing it and although all of them have proven to be untrue, it was continued until very recently.

In the late 1930s, physicians began to focus on the problem of low birth weight, and an accident of war demonstrated the importance of maternal nutrition in this regard. In 1945, railroad workers in western Holland, anticipating an imminent allied invasion, went on strike. The invasion did not come and the Nazis retaliated by imposing an embargo on transports into western Holland. Almost no food came in, and the winter of 1945 in Rotterdam and other cities in western Holland has since been referred to as the "Hunger Winter." The famine conditions lasted for nine months, until the allies liberated the country. However, the efficient Dutch hospital system had kept records of all deliveries during the famine, and these indicated that women who were pregnant during that time gave birth to infants one-half pound lighter on the average than those born to mothers before or after the famine or to mothers who lived in eastern Holland where food was available.

More recent studies, in developing countries, demonstrate even more dramatically the relationship between maternal nutrition and infant birth weight. For example, the birth weight in a poor population in Guatemala averaged one pound below that in more affluent populations. A food supplementation program was introduced, and within a year the difference disappeared. More careful analysis demonstrated that those women who, during their pregnancies, consumed at least 20,000 calories above their normal intake gave birth to infants within the normal birth-weight range. Interestingly, it did not seem to matter from what source those calories came, a point we will return to later.

Even from this short historical review, it is clear that the maternal diet has a powerful influence on fetal growth and birth weight. How, then, do we know when the mother's diet is adequate?

Weight gain during pregnancy The most important indication that a mother is consuming an adequate diet is that she is gaining enough weight during pregnancy. As we have seen, maternal weight gain during pregnancy correlates directly with infant birth weight, and in any population of pregnant women, those who gain more weight generally have bigger babies. But how much weight gain is enough? There are several ways of calculating this. The first is to simply watch "mother nature." In populations with abundant food and no restrictions on its consumption, women gain from twenty-five to thirty pounds during pregnancy. If this seems like a lot, some simple arithmetic will show how it accumulates. As we have seen, your blood volume during pregnancy will increase by about two and a half pounds, your uterus by about three pounds, and your breasts by two to three pounds, besides which you must deposit between ten and fifteen pounds of lactation fat. Taken together, this means that your own weight gain should range from eighteen to twenty-three pounds. Your fetus should weigh about eight pounds, the amniotic fluid about one pound, and the placenta another pound—a total of about ten pounds for the fetal component of your pregnancy. Thus, simple addition gives a twenty-eight to thirty-three pound weight gain. Because of these considerations, the American College of Obstetrics and Gynecology and the National Academy of Science have both recommended that a woman who is near her ideal weight before pregnancy should gain from twenty-five to thirty pounds during her pregnancy.

As you can see, nature, when left to its own devices, does very well.

Despite the need to gain weight over the course of your pregnancy, this gain should not be evenly distributed, but should be divided into a total gain of two to five pounds during the first trimester and three to four pounds per month thereafter. This pattern of weight gain will permit the proper changes to take place within your body at the proper time, will ensure proper placental growth, and will supply enough fuel for adequate development of your infant.

Your weight before pregnancy In the last chapter, I mentioned that one of the most important preparations for pregnancy is to bring your weight as close as possible to its ideal. If you are significantly underweight when you become pregnant, you will have to gain more weight during pregnancy to make up the deficit and properly support the growth of your fetus. Recent studies suggest that your body attempts to reach a weight after delivery that is about 110 to 120 percent of your ideal weight, and that if it reaches this weight, the growth of your fetus will be normal, whereas if it does not, your infant's birth weight will be below normal.

Figure 1 depicts the relationship between infant birth weight and the mother's weight after delivery in terms of a percentage of her ideal weight. As you can see, the weight of the infant increases until the mother reaches 110 to 120 percent of her ideal weight. At this point your infant will have attained his or her growth potential, and any further weight gain during your pregnancy will not produce any further fetal growth. This also means that if you are underweight before becoming pregnant, you will have to make up the deficit besides gaining the twenty-five to thirty pounds that are necessary for your pregnancy itself. This is not always easy to do, and if you are very underweight, the large amount of weight you will have to gain may be such that other problems could occur. Clearly, then, it is best to correct the deficit before becoming pregnant.

FIGURE 1

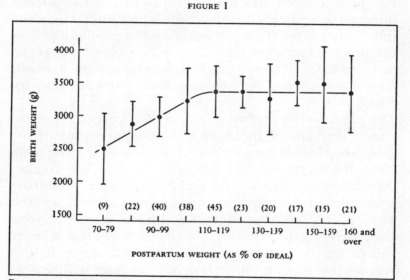

Postpartum weight, expressed as percent of ideal body weight and mean birth weight in 254 primiparas and multiparas. Values are mean ± S.D. Numbers in parentheses represent number of subjects.

From: P. Rosso, "Prenatal Nutrition and Fetal Growth Development," Pediatric Annals, Vol.10, No.11, November, 1981.

What if you are above your ideal weight before pregnancy? Unfortunately, the body of an overweight mother is not as efficient in dividing available nutrients between her and her fetus as that of an underweight mother. Perhaps this is because overweight, in terms of evolution, is a relatively new problem, and nature has not yet had a chance to adapt to it. Whatever the reason for this inefficiency, a mother who is twenty-five to thirty pounds overweight cannot afford to go through her pregnancy without gaining some weight, even though she can afford to gain somewhat less weight than a woman of normal weight. It appears that no matter how much a woman weighs before she becomes pregnant, she must gain at least fifteen pounds.

The effects of undernutrition on pregnancy We have seen that the birth weight of infants decreases when food is limited, and returns to normal when food becomes available. The major reason for this is that when food is scarce, the mother's body will actually hoard nutrients at the expense of the fetus, in order to be able to make them available after the infant is born. How does this happen? Recent studies with both animals and pregnant women have begun to uncover at least part of the answer.

As we saw earlier, the mother's body must make certain adaptations for her pregnancy to proceed normally. Furthermore, each adaptation depends to some degree on others that have taken place before. One of the earliest of such adaptations is the expansion of the maternal blood volume that provides blood for the developing uterus and placenta so that these organs can establish an adequately functioning pipeline between the mother and her fetus. It appears that when the mother's diet does not provide enough energy, the increase in her blood volume will be inadequate and the development of the fetal pipeline will be impaired. Under these conditions, the growth of the fetus will also be impaired; it will not be able to extract the nutrients it needs from the mother's blood. Only when enough calories are available can the fetus get the nutrients it needs regardless of whether those nutrients come from the mother's diet or from the breakdown of the mother's tissues. Currently available evidence points to a deficiency in calories as the cause of inadequate expansion of the maternal blood volume. When calories—and the energy they provide—are supplied in the mother's diet, her blood volume will expand normally, and the rest of the changes necessary to establish the fetal pipeline will take place.

The quality of your diet During pregnancy you should increase your caloric intake by three hundred to five hundred calories per day. This is not really very much; six ounces of meat alone contains three hundred fifty calories, a slice of toast contains sixty-six calories and a glass of milk contains one hundred sixty calories. Even an apple contains ninety-six calories. The appetite increase that normally accompanies pregnancy will ensure that you do this; if you eat when you are hungry and stop when you are satisfied, you will get enough calories.

However, you will need other foods besides those that provide calories. For example, although the evidence is incomplete, it appears that a proper proportion of carbohydrate, protein and fat in your diet is important, for while your body will adapt well to pregnancy as long as enough calories are available, your fetus requires large amounts of amino acids—the components of protein—to build its tissues. As we have seen, the placenta extracts these amino acids from your blood. They can get into your blood either from the protein in your diet—and during pregnancy the dietary protein requirement increases from 44 to 74 grams per day—or, if your diet is low in protein, as a result of the breakdown of your own tissues, especially your muscle tissue. Therefore, especially if your diet before pregnancy is not high in protein, your tissues may become depleted and your fetus may grow poorly. This situation is rarely seen in the United States because of the relatively high-protein diet we consume, but it is quite common in certain developing countries where the dietary protein content is low and pregnancies often come in rapid succession.

Despite the generally adequate protein content of the American diet, an exception occurs among pure vegetarians who eat no meat or meat products and no eggs. Most people who follow such a diet know that it is potentially low in protein and that they must be sure to eat certain plant foods such as rice and beans within a single meal in order to get all of the amino acids their bodies need. Therefore, a strict vegetarian who becomes pregnant should continue this practice and also take in the extra three to five hundred calories she needs from various foods rather than in the form of pure carbohydrate. Moreover, since vitamin B_{12} is present only in meat and meat products, she should take supplements of this vitamin. If she follows these and a few other simple rules (which we will discuss below), there is no reason for even the strictest vegetarian to discontinue such a diet during pregnancy. On the other hand, more restrictive diets, such as the Zen Macrobiotic diet, should be avoided. They are not only too low in calories but also deficient in almost every other essential nutrient, and can be dangerous even if followed for only a short time during pregnancy.

Specific nutrient requirements If your diet contained a wide variety of foods before pregnancy, simply increasing their quantity during pregnancy will help to ensure that you get all of the essential nutrients you need. However, while the requirements for all nutrients increase, the need for some increases more than for others, and it is the need for those nutrients normally in shortest supply in our diets that increases the most. These include iron, calcium, zinc and folic acid.

Making new blood Both iron and folic acid are essential for the body's manufacture of new blood cells. All cells, and particularly young red blood cells, need folic acid in order to be able to divide and so give rise to new cells, while iron is an integral component of the mature red cell. Vitamin B_{12} is also necessary for young red cells to divide. Fortunately, it is abundant in nature in all meat and meat products, and is stored in the body over long periods of time. In fact, a normal adult usually has stores of this vitamin that are adequate for an average of 2,000 days. Even though a woman's requirement for vitamin B_{12} increases by 25 percent during pregnancy (from 3 to 4 micrograms per day), her reserves should be more than adequate to meet her own and her fetus's needs. Strict vegetarians, whose diets are devoid of vitamin B_{12} and who may not have large reserves of this vitamin, should take a supplement of at least 4 micrograms per day.

Because the placenta distributes folic acid to the fetus in large amounts even if the mother's supply is low, and because this vitamin is not stored in the body, it must be constantly replenished. It is found in most meats, many fruits and vegetables, and certain legumes and grains (Table 6, page 87). Normally, the fetal blood contains two and a half times as much folic acid as the maternal blood, but this difference may be much greater if the mother is deficient in the vitamin. Only if the deficiency in the mother is very severe is the fetus unable to extract adequate amounts from the mother's blood, a situation that rarely occurs, and folic acid deficiency is rarely seen in infants. On the other hand, it is estimated that from 2.5 to 16 percent of all pregnant women have a folic acid deficiency, depending on the criteria used and the population studied. If you are consuming enough food to satisfy your need for calories, and if your choices include generous amounts of foods rich in folic acid, you probably do not need a folic acid supplement. However, since the need for folic acid doubles during pregnancy, from 400 to 800 micrograms per day, many physicians prescribe a supplement just to be sure. There is no danger in this, and it is a useful form of "insurance." The important thing to remember is that this is a supplement, and that the best source of folic acid is a varied diet.

Of all nutrients, the requirement for iron goes up the most during pregnancy. The need for iron increases both because the fetus is developing an entirely new blood supply and each of its newly formed red cells must contain iron, and because of the mother's need for an increased blood volume. After delivery the iron that the fetus and placenta have accumulated will be lost to the mother, and her own blood volume will return to normal. Since the body makes adaptations that let it take in more iron during pregnancy, you have the potential to come out of your pregnancy in a better iron status than you went into it with.

Figure 2 is a diagram of the body's iron requirements before, during and after pregnancy. As you can see, the need for iron decreases as you stop menstruating and does not increase significantly until the end of the first trimester. If you begin pregnancy with a reasonable amount of stored iron you will be at a decided advantage, and if your diet is rich in iron or if you take an iron supplement your stores can be further enriched.

As Figure 2 shows, your iron requirements increase rapidly beginning at about the tenth week of pregnancy, first to sustain the increase in your own blood volume and then to sustain your fetus. Before your pregnancy is over you will need to take in about 1,000 milligrams of extra iron, half of which (500 milligrams) will be lost at delivery. If your initial iron stores were low and you do not take a dietary iron supplement, you are at risk for becoming progressively depleted of iron as your pregnancy proceeds. This will probably have little effect on your fetus, since the

FIGURE 2

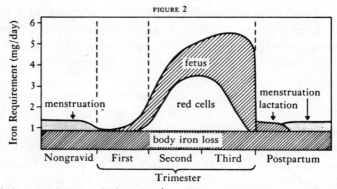

Daily iron requirements during pregnancy. These requirements are needed to meet the normal losses from the body and to provide iron for the enlarging red cell mass, the fetus and for lactation after the birth of the child.

From: T. H. Bothwell and R. W. Charlton, "Iron Deficiency in Women," A Report of the International Nutritional Anemia Consultative Group *(Washington, D.C.: The Nutrition Foundation, 1981), p.8.*

placenta will still do its job, preferentially distributing iron to the fetus; even severely iron-depleted mothers usually will give birth to infants whose iron status is normal. However, under these circumstances, the progressive depletion of iron from your body can cause symptoms of iron deficiency, including tiredness, weakness, irritability, restlessness and a loss of your attention span—a very undesirable situation when you are trying to adjust to being pregnant. In fact, many of these symptoms, which in the past were ascribed to pregnancy itself, are now known to be due to iron deficiency.

But while iron deficiency is quite common in American women (30 percent of whom are iron deficient before entering pregnancy), it need not happen to you. If you are in doubt about your iron status, ask your physician to check it. Before becoming pregnant, you can ensure that you have adequate iron reserves by consuming a diet rich in iron or by taking a supplement. If your iron stores are good when you become pregnant, continue to build them up during the first trimester by consuming iron-rich foods. If your stores were not built up, begin taking an iron supplement as soon as you know you are pregnant.

Although women who have good reserves and continue to consume an iron-rich diet during pregnancy probably need no supplementation, most American physicians routinely prescribe iron supplements during pregnancy. In view of the very high incidence of iron deficiency in American women, I have no objection to this practice. But, as with folic acid, such supplementation does not replace the need for an iron-rich diet. One reason for this is that foods rich in iron are also rich in other nutrients that are required in greater amounts during pregnancy and which an iron pill will not provide. Perhaps the most important of these other nutrients is zinc.

Zinc has recently been recognized as a very important trace mineral, particularly during such periods of rapid growth as pregnancy. There are several kinds of evidence for the importance of this nutrient. First, the placenta selectively extracts zinc from the maternal blood for its own growth and the growth of the fetus. As a result, the concentration of zinc in the blood of the fetus—like that of folic acid—is much higher than in the mother's blood. We have already seen that the placenta does this only when the fetal requirement for a nutrient is particularly high. Second, zinc deficiency in pregnant animals results in retarded fetal growth and a variety of birth defects. Third, low zinc levels in the maternal blood and amniotic fluid have been correlated with poor fetal growth in several human populations.

Zinc is found in many of the same foods as iron, and women who are iron deficient also tend to be zinc deficient. However, iron supplementation will not alleviate the zinc deficiency, and it is important to eat iron-rich foods as sources of zinc. The dietary solution to iron deficiency therefore provides a double benefit.

Building strong bones Earlier, we discussed the changes your body undergoes during pregnancy in order to take in more calcium. Your kidneys and placenta manufacture increased quantities of the vitamin D hormone (dihydroxycholecalciferol) that promotes calcium absorption. Your gastrointestinal tract absorbs more calcium, which the placenta preferentially carries into the fetal blood, where it is rapidly deposited in the fetal skeleton.

Just as with iron, the fetus will get its calcium regardless of how much you consume in your diet. If your intake is low your bones will release calcium into your blood to supply the fetus, which can create serious problems for you in later life in the form of osteoporosis (see Chapter 8). So, although nature has supplied you with the means to absorb calcium, you must take advantage of this by consuming enough calcium to maximize its absorption (about 1,200 milligrams per day). This is only one third more than your prepregnancy needs, and can be achieved easily if your diet is rich in dairy products such as milk, skim milk, cheese and yogurt. If for some reason you do not consume these products, a calcium supplement (500 milligrams per day) is appropriate. If you follow these simple principles, you should be able to supply your infant with sufficient calcium while at the same time preventing any calcium loss from your bones. Some recent studies even suggest that if you follow these rules you may finish pregnancy with a net gain of calcium in your bones.

Too much may not be good Fortunately, only a few of the nutrients required during pregnancy can be toxic to the fetus if taken in very large amounts. The two most important of these are vitamin A and vitamin D. There is also some evidence that large amounts of vitamin C in the maternal diet during pregnancy can produce problems for an infant after birth.

In very large doses, vitamin A causes malformations in

animals, and several cases of birth defects have been reported in the infants of mothers who ingested large doses
of this vitamin during pregnancy. It appears that the toxic
dose is very high and the problem is therefore quite rare.
By contrast, fetal toxicity from excess vitamin D during
pregnancy is a more widespread danger. In the late 1950s,
when I was still a young physician completing my resi-
dency, reports began to appear in British medical journals
of children being born with a syndrome of multiple birth
defects. But even though doctors in the United States were
on the alert for such infants, we did not see any, whereas
growing numbers of cases were being seen in England. The
cause took several years to identify.

Because of vitamin deficiencies during World War II, the
British had begun a massive vitamin fortification program
when the war ended; part of this program was the fortification of milk and many other staple foods with much larger
quantities of vitamin D than were used in the United
States. Furthermore, doctors actively encouraged vitamin
supplementation during pregnancy. The result was that in
some mothers, vitamin D accumulated to toxic levels, permanently damaging their fetuses. As soon as the cause was
discovered, the vitamin D fortification was reduced and
routine vitamin supplementation during pregnancy was
discontinued. The number of babies with deformities
caused by the vitamin then decreased dramatically and
soon practically disappeared. The moral of this story is that
if you are taking vitamin supplements during pregnancy,
don't take one that contains vitamin D.

A much less dramatic but also potentially serious problem may occur among women who consume very large
doses (from one to ten grams daily) of vitamin C during
pregnancy. Experiments in guinea pigs (one of the few
mammals other than humans and apes that requires vitamin C) have shown that the feeding of large doses of this

vitamin to the mother during pregnancy may result in offspring that have an increased capacity to break down the vitamin, and who therefore require greater amounts of it after birth. Although this dependency disappears if the pups are supplied with larger amounts of the vitamin, they can develop scurvy (a disease caused by vitamin C deficiency) and die if they get no vitamin C. A few case reports suggest that a similar problem may occur in humans, and although it is certainly not very common—since there would be many cases in view of the large number of people who now take large doses of vitamin C each day—it is something to be aware of if you are one of these people. Furthermore, there is no evidence that high doses of vitamin C offer any benefit during pregnancy. If you must take high doses of the vitamin, tell your obstetrician and pediatrician, so that they can watch your infant.

THINGS TO AVOID

Smoking As we have already noted, some aspects of your lifestyle may be particularly dangerous to your developing fetus. If you smoke, for example, your infant is likely to be smaller than he or she should be. Heavy smokers have babies that on the average weigh one-half pound less than babies born to women who do not smoke. The magnitude of the effect on the fetus is directly proportional to the number of cigarettes the mother smokes per day, and the fetus feels the effect of smoking throughout pregnancy. Therefore—and again—stopping or cutting down your smoking will benefit the fetus. One reason why some mothers say they fail in their attempt to give up smoking is that they gain weight rapidly. But since during pregnancy you want to gain weight rapidly, this may make it easier for you to stop or at least cut down. You owe it to your infant to try.

Alcohol The problem with alcohol during pregnancy is much different and potentially much more serious than that with cigarettes. It is also a problem that has been recognized for centuries. From the Bible we hear "Behold thou shalt conceive, and bear a son; and now drink no strong drink" (Judges 13:7)—a statement which, if taken literally, pinpoints the problem of alcohol and pregnancy. Alcohol can and does affect the human embryo from immediately after its conception. Moreover, even though you may not know you are pregnant, the embryo is already about six weeks old by the time you miss your second period. For the embryo, these early weeks are a time of enormous change. Its organ systems begin to develop, its specialized tissues are formed, and its cells rapidly divide and change in character and function. In fact most severe birth defects are caused by faulty development during this early embryonic period. It was during this period that thalidomide, a drug that caused tragic abnormalities, had its action against the fetus, and it is during this period that most drugs and other agents that cause deformities—including alcohol—act.

Recent evidence confirms earlier observations that a mother's consumption of two or more ounces of absolute alcohol per day (two mixed drinks, two five-ounce glasses of wine or two twelve-ounce cans of beer contain one ounce [30 milliliters] of absolute alcohol) may result in the group of malformations that have been named the "fetal alcohol syndrome." Although susceptibility to the syndrome varies, and there is little or no risk to the occasional drinker, many studies throughout the world, and particularly in the United States, have confirmed the dangers of heavy alcohol consumption early in pregnancy.

Such heavy drinking, besides resulting in abortion or severe birth defects, may also produce direct toxic effects on the embryo. Later, after the placenta and the fetus are formed, even moderate alcohol consumption, over a period of weeks or months, can reduce fetal growth and impair fetal brain development. Studies in animals and in human populations strongly suggest that prolonged, moderate alcohol intake results in a reduction in birth weight. Some studies even suggest that subsequent intellectual performance, as measured by I.Q. and other tests, may be impaired in children whose mothers consumed moderate amounts of alcohol throughout pregnancy. The mechanism by which these effects occur is being examined, and some evidence indicates that the placenta may be involved.

It is hard to understand why the danger of alcohol during early pregnancy has not been widely recognized or accepted until recently. Even in the mid-eighteenth century, when changes in the laws governing distillation led to the availability of large amounts of inexpensive alcoholic beverages in England, and that nation had a "gin epidemic," the Royal College of Physicians reported that mothers' drinking was "a cause of weak, feeble, and distempered children."

Later, in the nineteenth century, a committee of the British House of Commons, established to investigate drunkenness, concluded that infants born to alcoholic mothers had a starved, shriveled appearance. At the beginning of the century a mortality two and a half times greater than normal was reported in the infants of mothers who drank large quantities of alcohol.

In recent years more careful studies have again sounded the alert. Reports from France, a country with an annual per capita intake of sixteen liters of alcoholic beverages per year (the highest in the world), indicated that one out of every 312 infants born in that country was afflicted with the fetal alcohol syndrome. The frequency of abnormalities in the infants of heavy drinkers was found in French studies to be as high as 50 percent.

I have presented the evidence linking alcohol to impaired fetal growth and development in some detail, so that if the use of alcohol is an important part of your lifestyle, you can make your own decision about what to do.

However, I hope it is clear that in this discussion of alcohol I am not describing a situation that is at all similar to what occurs with poor nutrition or with smoking. In those cases fetal *growth* is affected by compromising the fetal pipeline. The ingestion of large amounts of alcohol affects fetal *development*, before the pipeline is actually formed.

Obviously, then, if you are a heavy drinker, you should do something about it before becoming pregnant. If you are a moderate drinker you will probably want to cut back as soon as you know you're pregnant. Some women who can change their habits easily might decide to abstain during pregnancy. This reduces the risk of the fetus's being affected by alcohol to zero, a situation that may give you more peace of mind.

Caffeine Studies in humans suggest that the consumption of large amounts of caffeine may cause abnormalities in fetal growth. Some studies even raise the possibility that infants whose mothers consume large amounts of caffeine during pregnancy may exhibit abnormal behavior soon after birth. However, these effects seem to occur only in cases where the mother ingests very large amounts of caffeine (eight to ten cups of strong coffee per day, or drugs which contain caffeine—some of which are sold over the counter). But even though the risk of these abnormalities appears to be much smaller than with smoking or alcohol, if you are a very heavy coffee drinker you may want to cut down during pregnancy. It is also a good rule to take no drugs during pregnancy without consulting your doctor. Drugs containing caffeine should be particularly avoided.

Practical tips Women sometimes experience nausea and

vomiting early in pregnancy. Although this is often referred to as morning sickness, it may occur at different times during the day. The symptoms may be very mild, but are sometimes quite severe. Here are some things you can do to reduce them:

> Make sure you are relaxed, comfortable and have fresh, odor-free air.
>
> If you feel nauseated soon after getting up in the morning, keep plain crackers at your bedside and eat a few before getting on your feet.
>
> Take smaller meals (even a few bites), and more frequent ones.
>
> Take liquids slowly and between meals.
>
> Eat lots of dry foods, such as bread.
>
> Generally, eat foods that *you* know are not unsettling, even though there is no set list of foods to eat or avoid, since foods well tolerated by some women are upsetting to others.

If these simple measures don't work, or if your symptoms persist beyond the third month of pregnancy, you should consult your doctor.

After this early period your appetite will increase, and eating should become fun. Let your appetite determine the amount you eat. Don't fight those urges for food—turn them to your advantage, for if used wisely they provide the route to proper nutrition.

Remember to gain the necessary twenty-five to thirty pounds during your pregnancy; approximately two to five pounds overall during the first trimester and about three to four pounds per month thereafter.

Choose foods that will provide not only calories but also the nutrients that are in shortest supply. For example, while five marshmallows and an ounce and a half of raisins both contain about one hundred twenty calories—or roughly one third the extra calories you need per day—the raisins contain more than twice the amount of protein, five times more calcium and three times more iron than the marshmallows. The raisins also have significant amounts of vitamin A and the B-complex vitamins, while marshmallows have none. As you can see, simply making the proper food choices will greatly increase your chances of getting adequate amounts of all the nutrients you need. This means taking the time to read labels and thinking about the foods you eat—a practice we should all develop but one that is particularly important during pregnancy. Remember too that variety is very important. It will ensure your supply of both the known important nutrients and those nutrients that we still know little about.

Finally, if you and your physician decide upon supplementation, the two most important nutrients to be supplemented are usually iron and folic acid. For those of you who can't or won't eat dairy foods, calcium can be taken in tablet form. If you are a strict vegetarian, vitamin B_{12} can also be taken in tablet form.

Table 1 is a simple guide to the daily food choices that will provide you with the necessary nutrients. This guide is certainly not the only way to achieve good nutrition during pregnancy. But for most of us who eat at least several foods from each of the groups in the table, it provides a practical means of consuming a varied and balanced diet during pregnancy.

There is nothing complicated about ensuring good nutrition during pregnancy. Nature has been doing it for millions of years. In fact, what little difficulty there is has been self-imposed by a lifestyle that emphasizes weight reduction and favors foods that are low in certain important nutrients. Pregnancy is a good time to let yourself go and follow your appetite. It is also the best time for you to temporarily (even perhaps permanently) alter certain as-

TABLE 1 NUTRIENTS FOR PREGNANCY—FOOD CHOICES

MAIN NUTRIENTS	FOOD GROUP	MINIMUM NUMBER OF SERVINGS
Protein and Iron	meat, fish, poultry, eggs, legumes/grains, nuts	4
Calcium and Protein	milk (all forms), yogurt, cheese	4
Vitamins A and C (fiber)	citrus and other fruits, leafy, red/orange and green vegetables, potatoes and other tubers	5
B Vitamins, Iron (fiber)	whole grain, enriched grain products (such as whole wheat products, enriched and fortified cereals)	4
Water (fluid)	juices, fruits, vegetables, beverages, water	6

From: M. Winick, Growing Up Healthy: A Parent's Guide to Good Nutrition. *(New York: William Morrow and Co., 1982), pp. 33–34.*

pects of your lifestyle, reducing or eliminating cigarette smoking and alcohol consumption and beginning to eat foods that contain an abundance of the nutrients necessary for your own good health and for the optimal growth and development of your expected baby.

So far we have discussed nutrition and pregnancy in the adult woman. However, there is one group of women to whom all of the nutritional principles that have been discussed are important, but who also have very special nutritional needs—the pregnant adolescent.

ADOLESCENT PREGNANCY

Adolescent pregnancy is more common in the United States than in any other industrialized country in the world. The number of infants born to American women 19 years old or younger is almost twice that in England, nearly three times that in France or Sweden and about 20 times greater than in Japan. Nearly one million American adolescents become pregnant every year, or one of every ten girls between ages 15 and 19. Of these, about 600,000 give birth, of whom about one quarter give birth again within one year.

Moreover, during the past decade, there has been an increase in the percentage of American teenagers giving birth. While in 1960 teenage mothers accounted for about 14 percent of all births, by 1977 that figure had risen to 17 percent. In that year, 42,000 babies were born to mothers under 16.

Many factors—biological, social and economic—have been responsible for this high rate of adolescent pregnancy in the United States.

During the past thirty-five years, the age of puberty among American girls has been decreasing steadily. Today the average girl reaches menarche at age twelve and a half, and about 13 percent of young girls begin to menstruate before they are eleven years old. Obviously this pattern of earlier menarche has resulted in a higher proportion of sexually mature adolescents, lengthening the time when a young woman is biologically capable of conceiving. Even more important to the growing number of teenage pregnancies may be the social and economic conditions that are now part of the fabric of life in inner city populations in the United States, where such pregnancy rates are highest.

Without doubt, the risk of complications of pregnancy is greater among adolescent mothers than in more mature women. They have smaller babies and hence a greater infant mortality rate. They also have a greater number of premature deliveries and cesarean sections (because of small pelvic outlets), and more frequently develop toxemia and anemia. What is unclear is how much of this increased risk is due to "biological immaturity" and how much is due to social and economic factors. Studies suggest that socio-economic factors play the dominant role in adolescents over fourteen years of age. In younger girls, "gynecologic age"—defined as the number of years since the beginning of menarche—plays the major role. A fifteen-year-old girl who began to menstruate at age twelve, for example, has the same biological capacity for a normal pregnancy as a woman in her late teens or early twenties. By contrast, a girl of fifteen who began menstruating at fourteen is more likely to have a complicated pregnancy.

Unfortunately, even though most adolescents who become pregnant are potentially capable of carrying their infants at very little increased risk, most do not, largely because of their environment and a lack of prenatal care and proper nutrition.

The nutritional requirements for the adolescent mother are the same as for the mature pregnant woman, but occur in addition to the requirements for her growth during this period of rapid change. Still, these requirements are often somewhat less than one might think, since the maximum rate of growth, regardless of the chronological age of a young girl, precedes menarche, and she will have passed her growth spurt before pregnancy can occur.

As we have seen, a normal adult woman should gain at least twenty-five pounds during pregnancy. A young woman who becomes pregnant two years after menarche would be expected to have gained three pounds in the next nine months if pregnancy had not ensued. Thus, besides the twenty-five pounds she needs to gain during pregnancy, she will have to gain three pounds for her own growth, or a total of twenty-eight pounds. Therefore, from the biological standpoint, the number of extra calories she will require will be minimal. Unfortunately, the problem is not quite so simple. Many pregnant adolescent girls come from socioeconomic environments that cause them significant nutritional deficiencies. The inner-city areas that produce most adolescent pregnancies, for example, also produce calorie, protein, iron and calcium deficiency, as well as folic acid and other vitamin deficiencies. Yet an adolescent mother who is ten pounds underweight before becoming pregnant will have to gain thirty-eight pounds during her pregnancy—not an easy job for anyone, and particularly difficult for an adolescent who may have erratic eating habits, mixed feelings about her pregnancy, and no economic ability to buy an adequate diet. The pregnant adolescent is therefore likely to have been suffering from nutritional deficiency before she became pregnant, which must be corrected during the pregnancy if her infant is to have the best possible chance of developing perfectly.

The pregnant adolescent is particularly at risk for a deficiency of iron, folic acid and calcium, since these three micronutrients, which are in shortest supply during pregnancy, are also in short supply during adolescence. A diet rich in iron, folic acid and calcium could fulfill this need, but is usually unavailable in such cases, and supplementation is therefore necessary. Thirty milligrams of iron, 500 mg of calcium, and 800 micrograms of folic acid per day should be taken as a supplement in addition to a high-calorie varied diet.

There have been few studies of adolescent mothers' ability to successfully nurse their infants without depleting themselves of vital nutrients. But as we shall see in the next chapter, lactation consumes many calories, and the diet of the adolescent mother must therefore be adequate both for the increased demands of lactation and for her own growth requirements. Calcium supplementation is particularly important in the lactating teenager (1 gm per day). The young, less mature adolescent should nurse her infant for a short time after birth, to give the infant the benefit of mother's colostrum, which is the first breast secretion and contains antibodies and other immune substances advantageous to the baby. Whether lactation should continue is a decision that the adolescent mother should make together with her doctor. It is important that both she and her infant grow properly. This may not always be feasible if the infant is totally breast fed, but may work quite well if it is partially breast fed. The young mother's wishes must be respected in this matter. It is her baby and her responsibility.

CHAPTER 6

The Nursing Mother

*F*or the mammalian infant, breast feeding is the bridge between an intrauterine existence and an independent life. Milk is the foundation of this bridge. It is the only food that, by itself, can provide all of the nutrients needed for adequate growth and development. And among the mammals, only a mother can produce the milk her infant needs. Moreover, no two mammalian milks are alike; each is tailored specifically to the infants of that species. In this chapter we will therefore describe the nutritional aspects of lactation, both from the standpoint that breast feeding is the best source of nutrition for the newborn and from the standpoint of the mother's nutritional needs.

COMPOSITION OF MAMMALIAN MILK

As we have already seen, pregnancy is the time during which the mother passes the raw materials of growth to her fetus through the placenta, and the fetus converts these materials into energy and the tissues of its body. After birth, the process is reversed; it is now the mother who manufactures a complete food from the raw materials in her diet, and the newborn infant who breaks this food down for energy or for the building of new tissue. Lactation is therefore much more of an energy-consuming process than pregnancy, and whereas you are likely to finish pregnancy with a net gain in weight, you are likely to complete lactation with a net weight loss. In fact, you will expend more energy during lactation than during any other period of your life.

If we assume that a mother uses her own energy very efficiently as she converts it to milk, it takes at least one calorie to make one milliliter of milk, or approximately thirty calories to make an ounce. Also, if your infant is fully breast fed, you will produce about six hundred milliliters or twenty ounces of milk per day. You will therefore expend at least six hundred calories per day in milk production alone. Is it any wonder that the calorie cost of breast feeding has been compared to "climbing Mount Everest"?

The calories in breast milk are divided among the three major nutrients; carbohydrate, fat and protein. The carbohydrate in human breast milk is a simple sugar called lactose. Since milk is practically the only source of lactose, and since this sugar is the major carbohydrate in the milk of nearly all mammals, it appears that lactose offers the young infant some advantage over other carbohydrates, although the exact nature of this advantage remains unknown.

The major source of calories in all milk is fat. In human milk, for example, fat provides about 50 percent of the calories. This makes milk an extremely calorie-dense food —since fat is the most concentrated source of calories—and permits the mother to provide her infant with large numbers of calories in a relatively small volume of fluid. On the other hand, the kind of fat in the milk of different mammals varies considerably. The fat in human milk, for instance, is much less saturated than the fat in cow's milk. Again, however, the significance of this is unknown.

Like carbohydrate and fat, the protein in milk can be used as a source of calories when energy is unavailable from other sources. However, the primary purpose of this protein is to provide the amino acids that the newborn infant requires for the synthesis of its new tissue proteins. Moreover, the rate at which infant mammals of different species grow and therefore lay down new protein is different, and this difference is reflected in the protein content of the mother's milk. As a rule, the faster the infant must grow, the higher the protein content of the mother's milk. The human infant grows relatively slowly, and human milk is therefore a relatively low-protein milk, containing about 1 percent protein. Cow's milk contains four times this amount and rat's milk twelve times as much. As in the case of calories, this has important ramifications as far as your own nutrition is concerned. In order to supply the amount of protein that should be present in a day's output of milk (six grams), you will have to take in about six grams more than your usual daily requirement (fifty grams of protein instead of forty-four). Since most American women consume well over fifty grams per day of protein even when not lactating, there is ordinarily no need for an increased protein intake during this period. By comparison, while half of the calories in a mother's diet are converted to fat during lactation, all of these calories are "lost" in the milk. As we shall see, the relatively small increase in the mother's protein requirement as compared to the large increase in her calorie requirement during lactation allows a certain amount of dietary flexibility during this time that is not so permissible at any other time in her life.

Although the quality of the protein is very high in all mammalian milks, each species manufactures a protein that is unique and highly adapted to the young infant of that species. The protein in human milk provides the optimal amounts of those amino acids that the human infant requires. No infant-formula manufacturer has been able to duplicate this protein. Instead, most infant formulas use protein derived from cow's milk as a substitute. Protein derived from soybeans has also been used under special circumstances, and in some countries protein derived from eggs or fish has been tried. But while all of these are useful under the proper conditions, none provides for the needs of the human infant as well as the protein manufactured in its mother's breasts.

As I mentioned at the beginning of this chapter, any infant mammal can survive and grow well for a short period after birth with its mother's milk as its only source of food. In the case of the human infant this period ranges from four to six months after birth, and its mother's milk must therefore contain adequate amounts of all of the nutrients the infant requires during this time. This includes all the vitamins and minerals it needs to grow and develop properly. But while the rapidly growing infant requires relatively more of almost all of the vitamins and minerals than the adult, the absolute amounts of these are quite small. What this means is that although the infant's requirements may be three times those of an adult on the pound-for-pound basis of body weight, the number of calories it will consume may be only 15 to 20 percent of the adult amount, since it weighs much less. Therefore, for most of the vitamins and minerals, the mother must make only a relatively small increase in her overall intake, which is easily accomplished by the increased appetite and food intake that normally accompanies lactation.

On the other hand, the breast milk is specially formulated so as to meet the infant's requirements for those vitamins and minerals that it requires in high quantities. The two most important nutrients in this regard are iron and calcium. Because of the huge demands for iron during pregnancy, both the mother and the infant enter the lactation period being vulnerable to iron deficiency. However, nature has given human milk a low iron content that allows the mother to hoard what iron stores she has left from pregnancy, leaving room for her to replenish these stores immediately after delivery. Moreover, the small amount of iron in breast milk is in a very highly absorbable form, permitting the newborn infant to absorb more than 30 percent of it, whereas she or he absorbs a much lower percentage of the iron in formulas made from cow's milk. For this reason, breast-fed babies rarely if ever become iron deficient, whereas formula-fed babies may need iron supplementation unless the formula is fortified. Exactly how the iron in breast milk is held in this easily available form is still a mystery.

Lactation makes calcium available to the newborn infant in several ways. First, all milk contains large amounts of calcium, and human milk is no exception. Second, the amount of calcium in human milk is about equal to that of phosphorus, which is optimal for calcium absorption. Third, the infant can absorb calcium extremely efficiently in early life. Current evidence suggests that this absorption occurs without the help of either vitamin D hormone or vitamin D in the mother's diet. In order to protect her bones, the mother also absorbs calcium very efficiently. The mechanism by which this is accomplished appears to resemble the one that works during pregnancy: the mother's kidneys make extra amounts of the vitamin D hormone, which then stimulates her gastrointestinal tract to absorb more calcium.

Thus, while the mother's iron requirement does not necessarily increase markedly during lactation (unless her stores are low), her calcium requirement does. In fact, the calcium requirement during lactation is higher than at any other time in adult life, and if this requirement is not met, the mother's bones will supply the calcium in her milk. Lactation is therefore a time when the mother is vulnerable to calcium depletion.

By now it should be clear that lactation, like pregnancy, is a unique time in a woman's life. It is not only a time of close emotional bonding to her infant, but a time when she will expend large amounts of energy to manufacture the nutrient-rich milk that will sustain her infant until it can begin to eat of its own accord. To produce and sustain the delivery of this milk the human breast must undergo several changes, some of which are begun by the mother's own body and others by her infant.

THE PRODUCTION AND DELIVERY OF BREAST MILK

There are three periods in every woman's life cycle when her breasts show marked development: adolescence, pregnancy and immediately after delivery. In all of these the breasts are preparing for their production of milk and its delivery to the infant. During adolescence, structural changes take place that create the architecture of the mature breast. By the time her adolescence ends, a young woman's breast consists of about twenty compartments or lobes, each of which is connected, by a tubelike duct, to a centrally located milk sinus or reservoir. The sinuses, which are located in a circle under the brown-pigmented area surrounding the nipple (the areola), are simply enlargements in the ducts that drain each lobe. Leaving the sinuses, the ducts narrow again, ending in openings that are visible on the nipple tip.

Each of the twenty-or-so lobes of the mature breast is further divided into smaller units called lobules; these contain several small sacs (alveoli) lined by the cells that produce the milk and expel it into the sacs. Muscle-like cells surround both the sacs and the small ducts that lead from them, squeezing the sacs and so forcing the milk down the ducts, into the reservoirs and out of the nipple openings.

Fat and connective tissue support all of these structures of the breast, and it is the amount of this supporting tissue, rather than the amount of glandular, milk-producing and delivering tissue that determines the size and shape of the breast. With few exceptions all women have enough glandular tissue to adequately nurse their infants.

Yet while all of this apparatus for milk production exists by the time a girl has passed through puberty, it is activated only during pregnancy and does not become fully functional until an infant begins to nurse at the breast.

As we have seen, the breasts enlarge during pregnancy as their blood supply increases. At the same time, under the influence of hormones produced by the mother and the placenta, the glandular tissues of the breast begin to prepare for milk production. The first substance they produce is the colostrum, the thick yellow liquid that is rich in antibodies and other proteins to protect the infant against disease, and which constitutes the bulk of the breast secretion for the first few days of nursing.

True lactation begins with several hormonal changes that take place as pregnancy ends. If adequate milk production is to continue, however, the infant must actually suck at the breast, stimulating two reflexes that maintain this production. The first reflex involves nerves that carry the suckling stimulus from the breast to the pituitary gland in the mother's head, prompting the latter to release the hormone prolactin. Traveling through the mother's blood, this hormone reaches the cells of the milk sacs, causing them to produce milk. The mother's production of milk therefore depends largely on how often and how well her infant sucks. The more often it sucks during the early days of breast feeding, the more milk she will produce. The milk supply will steadily increase when the infant is fed from both breasts at each feeding, and when nursings are frequent. Repeated suckling is so important that women who have not borne a child for a long time can be induced to lactate by having the infant stimulate the nipple and areola with repeated sucking. This is how the "wet nurses" in the past were so successful. Today some women who adopt infants have been able to initiate lactation in this manner and to nurse their infants successfully.

The second important reflex for continuing milk production is the so-called "let-down" reflex. It is concerned not with milk production but with milk release from the glandular tissues of the breast, and the ejection of this milk through the nipple pores into the infant's mouth. The let-down reflex is triggered by a variety of stimuli, including the infant's crying or the mother's sight or even thought of the infant, but again, the most important stimulus is the infant's suckling. Perhaps more important than what causes the let-down reflex is what inhibits it: fear, pain, anxiety, embarrassment or depression can all do this.

Like the prolactin-releasing reflex, the let-down reflex begins at nerve endings in the breast, which then transmit impulses to the pituitary gland. When they reach the gland, these impulses cause it to secrete the hormone oxytocin, which prompts the muscle cells around the milk sacs and ducts to contract, forcing the milk out of the glands into the ducts, which carry it down to the nipple, where it is ejected. The mother will often feel a tingling sensation as the let-down reflex is initiated. When the infant is first put to the breast the let-down reflex may occur irregularly; shortly thereafter, however, it will occur regularly within the first minute after nursing begins.

If let-down does not take place, milk backs up in the system, the breasts become engorged and painful, and a vicious cycle can be initiated as the mother, because she is not releasing milk, first becomes anxious and then depressed. Failure to establish a regular let-down reflex is often an important cause of lactation failure. This is significant, because while more than 50 percent of today's mothers attempt to breast feed, many give up the practice within days or weeks, blaming this on an inability to produce milk that will satisfy their infant. This explanation is rarely if ever correct. Usually the mother is nervous or anxious, or is breast-feeding her infant improperly, inhibiting her let-down reflex. In such cases milk may be produced but is not being released, with the result being a frustrated infant and an even more frustrated mother.

If you wish to nurse, it is important that you succeed, and as we shall see in the next section, good nutrition can help you to do this.

THE MOTHER'S NUTRITION DURING NURSING

A proper maternal diet is more important to a mother than to her infant. Unlike the fetus, the nursing infant is a very effective parasite, and will deplete your body of its reserves of fat, calcium, and even protein if you do not maintain an adequate intake of these nutrients. This drain is probably most obvious in developing countries, where many women, after repeated pregnancies and nursings, literally appear emaciated. But while this extreme situation does not exist in the United States, depletion of particular nutrients can occur during lactation unless the mother consumes a good diet.

Earlier, I mentioned that you will expend about 600 calories per day in order to produce milk for your infant. You will also have stored ten to fifteen pounds of fat (30,000 to 45,000 calories) during your pregnancy to help meet this caloric expenditure. During nursing, your body takes both of these sources of calories into account. But even with the increased appetite you will experience you will not be able to supply all of the extra calories you need, and your fat reserves will therefore slowly be used up. As a result, most women who wish to return to their pre-pregnancy weight after nursing need not watch their calorie intake.

Within the extra five hundred calories per day that most women consume during nursing, it is relatively easy to get most of the nutrients needed in larger amounts during this period. For example, twenty grams of extra dietary protein per day are recommended for supplying the protein in a mother's milk and for repleting her own body. And since twenty grams of protein contain eighty calories, only about one-sixth of the five-hundred calorie per day extra intake during lactation needs to be in the form of protein. This is probably more than you need, particularly since your diet is already likely to have a high protein content. But if you are a vegetarian, you should pay particular attention to this recommendation for extra protein.

The same principle holds for most of the vitamins and minerals. Although the requirements for these increase during lactation, they are easily met within the extra calories being consumed during this time. Thus if your diet is varied, within the boundaries that we have been discussing throughout this book, all you need do is increase the amount of food you usually consume. Your own appetite will dictate the amount of that increase.

However, special attention must be paid to getting an adequate supply of the nutrients that are in short supply in the average American diet, in order to prevent your own system from becoming depleted of them.

During nursing, as at other times in a woman's life, the most important of these are iron and calcium, and recent information indicates that zinc falls into this category as well.

Yet while getting enough iron is particularly important

for women because of their higher iron requirements than men, the situation is considerably improved during lactation because only small amounts of iron are "lost" in the breast milk, and because menstruation, in which iron is lost in the blood, may remain absent during this time or be much lighter than normally. If you take advantage of this special situation, which exists only during lactation, you will, with your five-hundred extra calorie-per-day intake, be able to replenish your iron supply and build up your reserves for the years to come.

Although zinc has recently been found to be very important to the growing infant, breast milk contains relatively large amounts of this nutrient. It is therefore important that you get enough zinc to prevent your own body from becoming depleted of it. Because—as we have already noted—the same foods that are high in iron are usually high in zinc, you derive a double benefit by consuming iron-rich foods during nursing. Foods such as meats, which contain iron in the "heme" form in which it is best absorbed, will provide about two to three times as much readily available iron as foods that contain iron in other forms, such as vegetables and fortified foods.

It is often said that lactation will deplete calcium from your bones and that this is the price a mother must pay to provide enough calcium for her growing infant. This is not necessarily true. There is no question that lactation presents a potentially disadvantageous situation: you are manufacturing large amounts of a product that has a very high calcium content and that is being "lost" from your body. However, your system has taken great pains to minimize this loss. Moreover, your infant's system is particularly efficient in absorbing the calcium in your milk. But you must still protect yourself by consuming enough calcium to meet the needs of your own bones and other tissues, and your diet should therefore be constructed in a

way that promotes calcium absorption from your gastrointestinal tract. Thus, the extra five hundred calories per day
that you will consume during lactation should be calcium-
rich calories. Table 1, Chapter 8, lists foods that are good
sources of calcium, and their calcium contents.

Remember also to reduce the amount of phosphorus you
eat at the same meal in which you consume calcium, since
phosphorus interferes with efficient calcium absorption.
As we have already noted, meat is a major source of phosphorus, as are many carbonated soft drinks. You may therefore want to follow a meat meal by a fruit dessert, and have
milk or cheese, which are very high in calcium, as a snack
a few hours later. Finally, a very high protein diet promotes calcium loss. Thus, while you should consume
enough protein to meet your increased requirements, you
should limit this protein to about 15 percent of your caloric
intake.

Table 1 gives a series of suggested daily menus that in
2,700 calories (the number consumed by the average nursing
mother) will deliver your daily requirement of all essential
nutrients, and which are particularly high in iron, zinc and
calcium. These menus are simply examples of the wide
variety of choices that will permit adequate growth of your
baby, good nutrition for yourself and a steady return to your
prepregnancy weight during the time you are nursing.

DIETING WHILE NURSING YOUR INFANT

Standard nutritional teaching points out that the nursing
period is no time for you to lose weight. After all, your
infant is being fed from your body, and your diet must
therefore be adequate to supply the infant's needs. If your
diet is restricted the infant will suffer. Ironically, however,
this teaching was until recently coupled with the recommendation of strict weight control during pregnancy. The

TABLE 1   THE LACTATION DIET MENUS*

The following menus give specific attention to several aspects of dietary needs during lactation.

TOTAL CALORIES:	The 2,700 calorie level meets the recommended energy needs for lactation. The 2,200 calorie level offers a modest reduction to permit a modest but steady weight loss.
TOTAL CALCIUM:	All of the menus provide no less than 1,200 milligrams of calcium.
TOTAL PROTEIN:	All of the menus provide 100 to 120 grams of protein.
VARIETY:	The menus are planned around easily available and popular foods. Because of the need for calcium they include many versions of dairy products. However, at least 25 percent of the calcium is provided in non-dairy foods.
	There is also an emphasis on whole-grain products. Fruits are suggested as the major part of between-meal snacks.
	The menus also recommend non-caffeinated teas, fruit juices, seltzer or water for additional fluid demands.
	Meals and snacks are spread out to accommodate individual variations in hunger and appetite.
ABBREVIATIONS:	tbsp. = tablespoon tsp. = teaspoon b/m = butter or margarine oz. = ounce

*Compiled by Maudene Nelson, R.D.

2,700 Calorie Lactation Diet—Menu # 1

BREAKFAST   8 oz. 1% fat milk
2 slices whole wheat toast
1 tsp. butter or margarine
2 oz. melted cheese
1 cup strawberries
herb tea or water

SNACK   1 medium orange
1 piece gingerbread

LUNCH   ½ cup cottage cheese
2 small bran muffins
4 tsp. butter or margarine
1 fresh nectarine
lettuce, tomato and cucumber
1 tsp. oil (on salad)
12 oz. grape juice

SNACK   1 fresh large apple (in wedges)
2 tbsp. peanut butter
2 rice cakes (wafers)
12 oz. apple juice

DINNER   1 cup cabbage
⅔ cup carrots
1 slice whole wheat bread
3 tsp. butter or margarine
1 tsp. oil
3 oz. veal
1 cup tossed salad
8 oz. 1% fat milk

SNACK   1 fruit flavored yogurt
herb tea or water

2,700 Calorie Lactation Diet—Menu # 2

BREAKFAST   4 oz. pineapple juice
½ melon
1 cup oatmeal
1 tsp. butter or margarine

2,700 Calorie Lactation Diet—Menu # 2

8 oz. 1% fat milk
½ cup cottage cheese

SNACK
2 slices raisin bread
2 tsp. butter or margarine
12 oz. apple juice
2 medium peach halves

LUNCH
¾ cup carrot-raisin salad
2 slices whole wheat bread
2 tsp. mayonnaise
3½ oz. turkey
lettuce, tomato and cucumber
8 oz. grapefruit juice

SNACK
1 medium banana
12 oz. 1% fat milk

DINNER
1 cup peas and mushrooms
1 cup yellow squash
2 tsp. butter or margarine
1 cup tossed salad
1 tsp. oil
3 oz. flank steak (lean)
2 fig bars
herb tea or water

SNACK
6 oz. vegetable juice

2,700 Calorie Lactation Diet—Menu # 3

BREAKFAST
8 oz. 1% fat milk
1 blueberry muffin
1 oz. Canadian bacon
1 egg, scrambled
1 tbsp. butter or margarine
1 cup citrus sections

SNACK
4 graham crackers
1 fresh pear
herb tea or water

2,700 Calorie Lactation Diet—Menu # 3

LUNCH	½ cup cole slaw
	3 oz. lean beef pattie
	1 oz. cheese
	1 hamburger roll
	1 baked apple
	12 oz. apple juice
SNACK	8 oz. 1% fat milk
	1 cup fruit cocktail
	6 saltine crackers
DINNER	2 breadsticks (Vienna type)
	¾ cup chick peas, onion, green peas, tomato salad
	2 tsp. oil (+ vinegar in salad)
	4 oz. baked chicken
	1 cup spinach
	8 oz. 1% fat milk
SNACK	herb tea or seltzer
	2 cups popcorn (plain)

reasoning behind this was that the fetus was a parasite and would get what it needed from the mother even if her weight gain was strictly controlled, whereas the nursing infant depended upon the mother's milk supply, which was directly controlled by the mother's diet. A poor diet therefore meant a reduced quantity and quality of milk and poor infant growth. Today, the evidence points strongly in the exact opposite direction for both pregnancy and lactation.

We have already seen that during pregnancy the mother will continue to store calories in the form of fat even at the expense of fetal growth. Once you begin lactation, however, all available evidence suggests that you will produce the same amount of milk, of the same quality, even if your calorie intake is restricted. Only with severe and prolonged malnutrition will the quantity of your milk be reduced, and even then its quality will remain essentially unchanged.

Because this may sound like an extreme statement, let me give you some of the evidence on which it is based. Women in developing countries who are themselves malnourished can still nurse their infants successfully for the first few months, with these infants gaining as much weight in the first three to four months of life as those nursed in the most affluent societies. For example, even under the extreme deprivation of Japanese prison camps women were able to nurse their infants successfully. A few other studies in which direct measurements were made showed that women whose diets were low in calories produced the same amount of milk, with essentially the same composition, as milk produced by mothers under far more comfortable circumstances. Thus, calorie restriction will not affect the mother's milk supply or alter its quality. What it will do is deplete the mother's reserves, first by using up her fat stores and then (if the restriction continues) by using her lean tissues to supply the needed energy.

Theoretically, then, a mother's careful control of her caloric intake will still allow her infant to grow normally, as well as deplete her fat stores and result in effective weight loss.

From a practical standpoint, too, you may be very sure that your infant will tell you if he or she is not getting enough milk. Under such circumstances your infant may want to nurse more often, and will rapidly empty each breast. If the infant remains unsatisfied, its growth rate will slow down. Therefore, if your infant shows no signs of hunger and grows at the proper rate and if your breasts remain full, you can afford to limit your calories.

In fact, I suggest that if you are truly overweight you take advantage of the extra energy demands of the nursing period to safely feed your infant while losing some or all of your extra weight. Everything is working in your favor: first, you are expending 600 extra calories per day without exercising, an expenditure that would be almost impossible if you were not nursing. Second, your body has adapted in such a manner that you are conserving iron and absorbing calcium at maximum efficiency. Third, your growing infant helps you to make sure your diet is adequate. The one problem you are likely to have is with your increased appetite, meaning that you will have to exert a certain amount of "willpower" to make those pounds come off. The three-stage reducing diet I am about to suggest for women who are truly overweight and want to reduce while nursing should help satisfy the appetite while at the same time controlling calories.

Stage I—Follow your appetite During the first few weeks after your baby is born, your main concern should be to establish a firm nursing relationship with it. This is a time to get used to nursing and to be sure that your milk supply is ample and is being adequately delivered. It is no time to begin a diet. So follow your appetite—it will certainly increase—and try to take in your extra calories from a wide variety of foods.

Your next step, once you are comfortable and your infant is nursing well (usually after about two weeks), is to begin to observe carefully what you are eating. You may even want to keep a diary. Try to modify your diet so that it approaches the kind of diet suggested in the previous section—a diet that emphasizes iron, zinc, and calcium and is generally high in vitamins and minerals. Note, too, which foods in your diet are high in calories and low in other nutrients, the "empty" calorie foods. These are the first foods to eliminate when you begin controlling your calories.

Stage II—Calorie control When you have nursed for about two weeks and have carefully observed your eating pattern for another week (while assuring yourself that your infant is growing normally) you are ready to begin limiting your calories. Your first step is to cut your calories to 2,200—the normal requirement for most women who are not nursing. Since at this level you should still be expending about six hundred calories per day more than you are taking in, you should be able to lose about a pound and a half to two pounds per week. This means a weight loss of between twenty and twenty-five pounds in three months and more than thirty pounds in four months.

Your next step—since you have limited your calories— is to make sure that the foods you eat are nutrient-dense foods, very high in the essential nutrients. While the eating of such foods is the basic principle of any reducing diet, it is easier to achieve on this diet because you can consume more calories and hence more food. Pay particular attention to iron- and calcium-rich foods. Table 2 gives a basic 2,200-calorie-per-day menu plan that is particularly high in calcium, iron, and zinc and which has adequate amounts of all of the essential vitamins and minerals. This diet is also high in fiber, which will supply bulk without calories to satisfy your increased appetite. However, because of the increased requirements for iron and calcium during lactation, you should also consume an iron supplement (30 milligrams per day) and a calcium supplement (500 milligrams per day).

Keep a record of both your own weight loss and your infant's weight gain. Your pediatrician can give you charts on which this can be plotted. It is very satisfying and can be very exciting to see your infant steadily gaining weight while you steadily lose it. A particularly exciting time comes when you reach your prepregnancy weight and continue losing as you head down to the normal weight for your age and height.

Stage III—Back to maintenance When you reach your weight goal, or a few weeks before you decide to wean your infant—whichever comes first—you can slowly increase your caloric intake. With a daily intake of 2,200 calories, some women don't even feel they are dieting. If this applies to you, just keep at this level, and after weaning your infant you will be consuming just the right number of calories to maintain your new, slimmer body. On the other hand, some women find that they must exert a lot of willpower to stay on a 2,200-calorie-per-day diet. If this is your situation—and since the weaning period often causes anxiety in both mother and infant, it is wise to remove the added strain of the diet before actually beginning to wean your child. Follow the dictates of your appetite. It will gradually decrease as you wean your infant (abrupt weaning is never recommended). You can return to the diet after your infant is successfully eating on its own.

FOR MOTHERS WHO DO NOT BREAST FEED

Although more than half of all new mothers now breast feed for at least a short time, and this number is increasing steadily, the remainder still prefer to bottle-feed their infants. There is no question that an infant can be reared successfully on modern infant formulas, yet breast feeding offers important advantages to the infant both psychologically and nutritionally.

It also offers psychological and nutritional advantages for the mother. I have mentioned the two most important nutritional advantages of breast feeding in earlier sections of this chapter: the greater ease of repleting nutrients depleted during pregnancy, and a more rapid return to one's prepregnancy weight. Therefore, if you elect not to breast feed, you must pay even more attention to nutrition than a mother who nurses her infant.

To begin with, you will weigh ten to fifteen pounds more after the birth of your infant than you did before becoming pregnant. These extra pounds must be lost. Fortunately,

TABLE 2

2,200 Calorie Lactation Diet—Menu # 1

BREAKFAST	1 cup oatmeal 2 tsp. butter or margarine 6 oz. 1% fat milk ½ cup cottage cheese ¼ melon 4 oz. pineapple juice
SNACK	1 medium fresh banana 1 slice raisin bread 1 tsp. butter or margarine herb tea or water
LUNCH	8 oz. cream of tomato soup 2 tbsp. peanut butter 2 slices whole-wheat bread 1 tbsp. strawberry jam 1 tangerine herb tea or water
SNACK	1 medium fresh peach 8 oz. 1% fat milk
DINNER	1 cup spaghetti ½ cup tomato sauce 4 oz. lean meat balls ½ oz. parmesan cheese 2 cups tossed salad 2 slices Italian bread (20 grams) 1 tsp. butter or margarine 1 tsp. oil (on salad) herb tea or water
SNACK	1 fruit-flavored yogurt

2,200 Calorie Lactation Diet—Menu # 2

BREAKFAST	1 English muffin 3 tsp. butter or margarine 1 egg, scrambled

2,200 Calorie Lactation Diet—Menu # 2

	¾ cup sliced peaches 6 oz. apple juice
SNACK	1 medium orange 4 graham crackers herb tea or water
LUNCH	1 large pita 3 oz. salmon (include bones) 1 tbsp. mayonnaise (blended with salmon) lettuce, tomato and cucumber 1 medium apple 12 oz. tomato juice
SNACK	1 medium banana 8 oz. fruit-flavored yogurt herb tea or water
DINNER	8 oz. 1% fat milk 1 medium potato 1 cup kale 1 cup tossed salad 2 tsp. butter or margarine 1 tsp. oil (on salad) 4 oz. broiled chicken breast
SNACK	herb tea or water 4 oz. ice cream

2,200 Calorie Lactation Diet—Menu # 3

BREAKFAST	2 slices French toast 2 tsp. butter or margarine 1 egg ½ cup 1% fat milk ½ cup apple sauce herb tea or water
SNACK	½ grapefruit 2 sesame bread sticks herb tea or water

2,200 Calorie Lactation Diet—Menu # 3

LUNCH	2 slices bread
	3½ oz. turkey
	1 tbsp. mayonnaise
	2 medium plums
	7 oz. orange-grapefruit juice
SNACK	1 medium fresh pear
	¼ cup cottage cheese
	herb tea or water
DINNER	1 small dinner roll
	8 oz. 1% fat milk
	½ cup rice (parboiled or brown)
	1 cup broccoli
	1 cup tossed salad
	2 tsp. butter or margarine
	1 tsp. oil (on salad)
	2½ oz. broiled pork chop
SNACK	herb tea or water
	1 cup fruit flavored yogurt

the reduced appetite that follows delivery in mothers who do not nurse is often enough to bring their weight gradually back to its prepregnancy level. For many others, however, this is not enough, and a "weight problem" can develop. Many overweight women complain of an increased weight that began after their first pregnancy and became progressively greater with each subsequent pregnancy, while never associating this with a lack of nursing, which is its true cause. Far fewer complaints of this "postpregnancy" weight gain are heard from mothers who nurse their infants.

A second problem for the non-nursing mother is the abrupt post-delivery shut-off of the mechanisms that favor the absorption and preservation of various essential nutrients. We have seen how important these mechanisms are for iron and calcium maintenance. During nursing, for example, a woman's menstrual blood loss is minimal, whereas it rapidly returns to its pre-pregnancy quantities in women who do not nurse. This means that the woman who does not breast feed not only loses iron more rapidly than the woman who does, but that she also consumes less food to replace the iron depleted during pregnancy. The situation with calcium is much less clear. On the one hand the lactating woman "loses" a great deal of calcium in her milk, while on the other she is able to absorb calcium much more efficiently. Therefore we do not know whether the nursing or nonnursing mother is better off from the standpoint of preventing calcium loss from her bones. The current view is that both are at risk and that both must therefore pay special attention to meeting their calcium needs.

Thus, since pregnancy and lactation are really a continuum in many ways, the woman who chooses not to breast feed may interfere with nature's way of ensuring her body's return to its prepregnancy nutritional status. She must therefore pay particular attention to her nutrition immediately after delivery.

If you decide not to breast feed, you must first reduce your calorie intake to a level at or slightly below what it was before you became pregnant. Watch your weight loss as long as it continues, regardless of how rapidly you lose weight, and you will be all right. If you stop losing weight before you reach your prepregnancy weight, reduce your calorie intake slightly further. Don't try to lose weight too quickly. Doing so will mean having to cut your calorie intake considerably, which will make the repletion of your body's iron and calcium stores much more difficult. Do favor foods that have a high iron content, particularly those from animal sources, which are more efficiently absorbed (see Table 2, Chapter 1), and consume large amounts of foods with a high calcium content (see Table 1, Chapter 8), at meals or snacks in which you do not eat red meats or consume carbonated drinks. Also, because of the potential problem of shortages, I feel that all mothers who do not breast feed should take an iron (30 milligram per day) and a calcium (500 milligram per day) supplement for a few months. Strict attention to these three points should permit you to skip the nursing period while returning to a good nutritional status within a reasonable time after your baby is born.

In this chapter, I have tried to point out the opportunity that breast feeding provides to improve your overall nutritional status, despite the nutritional strain it puts on your system. But whether you elect to breast feed or not, you cannot simply ignore nutritional considerations. You must control your calories while consuming foods that are good sources of iron, calcium and the other essential nutrients for yourself and—if you nurse—for your infant. In either case, good nutrition in the period following pregnancy can significantly contribute to your future health and well-being.

CHAPTER 7

The Reproductive Years

*A*lthough we have discussed how a woman prepares for pregnancy and lactation, most women spend only a relatively small time within their reproductive years bearing or breast feeding a baby. Most of these years are spent in many other activities that have little if anything to do with these functions. Yet this same period, often the most productive and rewarding in a woman's life, still requires special attention to nutrition, both to make it a healthy time and to delay some of the changes that occur with aging.

Various physiological and hormonal processes unique to women during the reproductive years have important nutritional implications. For example, besides the loss and need for replacement of iron and other nutrients during menstruation, many women have premenstrual cramps and other discomforts that can affect their appetite and intake of food.

As important as these physiological factors are, the nutritional status of women during the reproductive years is influenced much more by their lifestyles. For over the past two decades, vast numbers of women have begun employing some form of contraception, using alcohol and other drugs such as tranquilizers, smoking and perhaps most important nutritionally, dieting. All of these factors operate together to make the adult American woman much more vulnerable to a variety of nutritional deficiencies than her male counterpart.

This combination of physiological processes and lifestyle often results in a gradual depletion of key nutrients during the reproductive years. And this is ironic, since it appears that nature intended these years to serve as a storage period for nutrients needed in the years after menopause, when some of them become less readily available to the body. Yet perhaps even more ironic is that the lifestyle and dietary changes of the past two decades have increased the life expectancy and increased the postmenopausal period in American women by more than twenty years, making the avoidance of nutritional deficiencies during the reproductive years essential.

In this chapter I will discuss the major physiologic and hormonal processes that put women at a potential nutritional risk during their reproductive period. We shall see how eating patterns and other aspects of a woman's lifestyle can increase that risk and, for some crucial nutrients, result in frank deficiency.

NUTRITION AND THE MENSTRUAL CYCLE

From puberty to menopause, a period of more than thirty years, every woman undergoes a monthly cycle involving hormones produced by her pituitary gland and ovaries, and the response to these hormones by the organs concerned with reproduction: the ovaries, uterus and breasts. Under the influence of FSH (Follicle Stimulating Hormone), a hormone secreted by the pituitary gland, the ovary prepares to release a mature egg cell while at the same time secreting two hormones of its own, estrogen and progesterone, which act on the uterus to prepare it for receiving the egg cell and on the breast tissues to prepare them for manufacturing milk should fertilization occur.

The egg cell is released from the ovary about halfway through the menstrual cycle, and begins its free-floating journey down the fallopian tubes into the uterus. It is at this time that many women experience pain, irritability and some loss of appetite ("Mittelschmerz"). All women also experience an increased temperature (by about one degree) when the egg cell is released. In fact, many doctors use this temperature increase to pinpoint the time of ovulation. Few people realize, however, that this increased temperature requires the expenditure of one hundred calories per day at a time when the discomfort of Mittelschmerz may reduce a woman's food intake.

Yet from the standpoint of a woman's overall nutrition, the time surrounding the menstrual period is much more important. If the egg cell is not fertilized, the uterus, which has prepared itself for a possible pregnancy by building up the tissues in its wall and by trapping blood in newly expanded blood vessels, suddenly begins to contract. Blood and tissue begin to be released and menstruation begins. The entire period may last from one to five days or more, often marked by cramps, severe headaches, fatigue, nausea and even vomiting. Many women are literally incapacitated for three or four days during each monthly period—a total of from 10 to 15 percent of their reproductive years.

For the woman whose periods are heavy and prolonged, the normally added nutritional demands of menstruation are often inadequately met. The result over a long time may be deficiencies in vital nutrients, affecting her health and depleting the reserves she needs for her later years.

If your periods are heavy and long you should be paying

particular attention to getting adequate supplies of iron, zinc, folic acid and protein. And if discomfort prevents you from consuming your usual diet before and during menstruation, you must take special precautions to eat foods rich in these nutrients during the rest of the cycle.

REPLACING YOUR LOSSES

The nutrient most depleted by menstruation is iron. Nearly all of this is lost in the menstrual blood, of which an average woman with a normal reproductive cycle will lose 15,000 milliliters (about 30 pints) over her reproductive years—or the equivalent of her entire blood supply every five years. Many women lose two or three times this amount, replacing their entire blood supply every two years. This translates into about 75 grams of iron (7,500 milligrams) lost between puberty and menopause, an amount that must be replaced in food.

Given this loss, it is no wonder why women are much more prone to iron deficiency than men, nor is there any wonder that statistics show up to half of all women in the United States suffering from some degree of iron deficiency.

The best way to replace the iron lost in menstruation is through a diet rich in iron, which—since foods rich in iron are often also rich in protein, zinc and folic acid, the other nutrients lost during menstruation—will also go a long way toward protecting you from deficiencies in these other nutrients. Remember, you do not have to replace the iron on the same day it is lost or even the next day. However, you will have to be compensated for each day in which your iron intake is low during the following days. If you simply cannot consume enough iron-rich food during your menstrual period, you must be even more careful during the rest of the cycle. To illustrate this, suppose that your menstrual periods last three days and are fairly heavy and that you cannot follow your normal diet from the day before you menstruate and the three days of your menstruation—a total of four days. You will have lost about twenty-five milligrams of iron, which you will have to replace in the twenty-four days before you begin to menstruate again.

Furthermore, since only 5 to 10 percent of the iron you consume will actually be absorbed by your body (depending on the source of the iron), you will have to take in an *average* of up to twenty milligrams of iron per day just to replace your iron losses during a single menstrual cycle. This is a greater amount of iron than the recommended daily allowance because the latter is calculated on the basis of daily iron consumption, and does not include the days during menstruation when you may not eat.

Table 2, Chapter 2, lists foods high in iron and the iron content of the usual portion of each food. Figure 1 shows the percent of iron absorbed from various types of food. A good general rule to remember is that your body absorbs from 10 to 20 percent of the iron in meat and from 5 to 10 percent of the iron in vegetables and other plant foods.

Whatever foods you eat, the following important point should always be kept in mind: the amount of iron you will be able to derive from your diet depends partly on the amount of food you take in. Thus, the lower your overall food intake the lower your iron intake. However, if your diet provides you with 1,800 or more calories per day, you should not have any difficulty in meeting your iron requirement. Just choose generously from the list in Chapter 2. On the other hand, if you are constantly watching your weight you may find it difficult to get enough iron in your diet, and if you are on a very-low-calorie (below 1,200) reducing diet it may be almost impossible.

There are two ways to solve the iron problem that comes

FIGURE 1

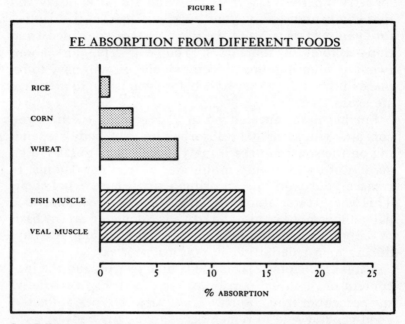

From: T. H. Bothwell and R. W. Charlton, "Iron Deficiency in Women," A Report of the International Anemia Consultative Group (INACG), (Washington, D.C.: The Nutrition Foundation, 1981), p. 12.

with a low-calorie diet. The first is to use foods, particularly cereals, that are fortified with iron. Such foods (if not pre-sweetened) have the advantage of being low in calories and relatively high in iron. You can enhance your absorption of iron from the cereal by taking a source of vitamin C (citrus fruits or juices) at the same meal. The second way to solve the iron/diet problem is to take an iron supplement. This is the least preferred method for increasing one's iron intake, but for women who have heavy periods, are constantly dieting or are vegetarians may be the only way of meeting their iron requirements.

Because the body has enormous protein reserves in its

various tissues, particularly in muscle, and because most American women consume far more protein than they need, the loss of protein is much less serious than the loss of iron through menstrual bleeding. Still, women who are strict vegetarians should pay particular attention to getting enough protein, especially if they lose large amounts of blood during their menstrual periods. We have already discussed protein "complementing" in the vegetarian diet by using plant foods whose amino acids, in combination, will supply all of the required amino acids. This is particularly important for vegetarians who lose blood heavily when menstruating.

Zinc and folic acid are the two other nutrients that may exist at low levels in women who repeatedly have heavy menstrual cycles. In contrast to iron or even protein loss, only very small amounts of these nutrients are actually lost during menstruation. Yet heavy bleeding means the loss of blood cells, which must be replaced by the manufacture of new bloods cells in the bone marrow, and both zinc and folic acid are required for this process. Furthermore, the more blood cells that are lost during menstruation, the greater the requirement for zinc and folic acid. Thus, women who menstruate heavily must take special care to ensure an adequate supply of zinc- and iron-rich foods in their diets.

Zinc is generally found in foods that are rich in iron. As we have already seen, this is one reason why it is far better to replace the iron lost during heavy menstrual bleeding with dietary sources of iron than with iron tablets. Folic acid is found mainly in leafy green vegetables, although certain meats such as liver are also good sources.

As with iron and protein, you will have a more difficult time meeting your zinc and folic acid requirements if you limit your food intake by dieting. And as with iron, a good source of zinc and folic acid can be fortified cereals. However, since the amount of these nutrients that manufacturers put into fortified foods varies widely from one brand to another, it is important that you check the labels carefully. The use of fortified foods may be particularly important if you are a strict vegetarian, since—as shown in Table 1, Chapter 2—the main source of zinc is animal products.

Although it is unusual, vitamin B_{12} deficiency can occur with heavy menstrual blood loss if no meat or meat products are included in the diet. Here again the loss of blood cells increases the requirement for this vitamin, which again, like zinc and folic acid, is needed for making new cells. However, since the normal daily requirement for vitamin B_{12} is very low, and since the vitamin is present in virtually all meat products, only the strictest vegetarians are susceptible to deficiency. If you fall into this category, you should use fortified cereals or vitamin B_{12} supplements.

REDUCING THE SYMPTOMS OF
HEAVY MENSTRUAL PERIODS

As we have seen, your monthly menstrual periods, particularly if heavy, can lead to nutritional deficiencies, partly through the loss of various nutrients, partly because of an increased need for other nutrients and partly because your food intake may be poor during menstruation. Obviously if these factors apply to you, you must try to alter them, both to prevent nutritional problems and to improve the quality of your life.

But what about the psychological and physical discomforts of menstruation that often cause such nutritional and other difficulties? Many remedies are used for this, some available at home and others prescribed by a physician. Perhaps most fall into the categories of pain relievers or tranquilizers. Yet while these remedies certainly have their place when the symptoms of menstruation are severe, you still pay the price of the side effects of these drugs, which may themselves be unpleasant.

Unfortunately, many women who do not wish to depend on drugs for relief of their menstrual discomfort, and therefore seek more "natural" methods, fall prey to all kinds of claims, many of which come under the heading of "nutritional cures." Through the ages, one or another type of nutrient has been recommended for relieving premenstrual and menstrual tensions. Today, high doses of certain vitamins seem to be in vogue. We read about the B vitamins thiamin or niacin, or the entire B-vitamin complex being used for this purpose; we hear about vitamin E in large doses and more recently about vitamin C in large doses. At one "health fair" I attended some years ago, single amino acids such as leucine or isoleucine were being heralded as cures for the symptoms of menstruation.

It would be wonderful if even one of these remedies worked; however, there is no scientific evidence of which I know that such remedies provide any improvement whatsoever. Furthermore, while many of them are harmless, others can have toxic effects. For example, high doses of nicotinic acid, a form of niacin, can cause flushing of the skin, burning sensations in the tips of the fingers and toes, and other unpleasant effects. High doses of vitamin A (which were advertised to cure premenstrual tensions in the past) can be extremely toxic and, if taken for long periods, can result in permanent disability and even death.

On the other hand, certain nutrient deficiencies may themselves aggravate the symptoms that accompany menstruation. Recently a deficiency of the trace mineral magnesium has been shown to have such an effect; in a study of the mineral, women who were magnesium-deficient had severe pain, anxiety, and fatigue during their menstrual periods. Magnesium supplementation reduced these symptoms in a significant number of the women. A varied diet could do the same thing, since the amount of magnesium supplement needed to reduce the symptoms in the study was within the range of the magnesium available in the normal diet.

Nevertheless, such studies are likely to be misinterpreted and even misrepresented, with the result that high doses of magnesium will soon be recommended for "curing" menstrual tension.

If you want to be sure that the lack of some nutritional factor is not aggravating the symptoms of your menstrual periods, eat an adequate and varied diet. If this still does not work, try a vitamin and mineral supplement. But do not fall for "instant remedies" that require you to use huge doses of this nutrient or that. They will surely cost you money, and may cost you even more by producing uncomfortable and dangerous side effects.

Nutrition does have one important, direct connection with menstrual abnormalities: Obese women have a higher incidence of irregular menstrual periods and very heavy bleeding during their periods than lean women. Several studies have demonstrated this direct relationship between the extent of obesity and such menstrual irregularity and blood loss. In simple terms, the fatter you are the more likely it is that your periods will be heavy and irregular. Obese women also show a tendency to have more facial hair and to have menstrual cycles more than thirty-six days long. Figure 2 demonstrates these relationships.

Nevertheless, while such studies have shown an association of obesity with such effects, they do not prove that obesity *per se* is the cause of the effects. Some people have argued that obese women are under more tension than those of normal weight, and that it is this tension that is responsible for their menstrual abnormalities. Others have

FIGURE 2

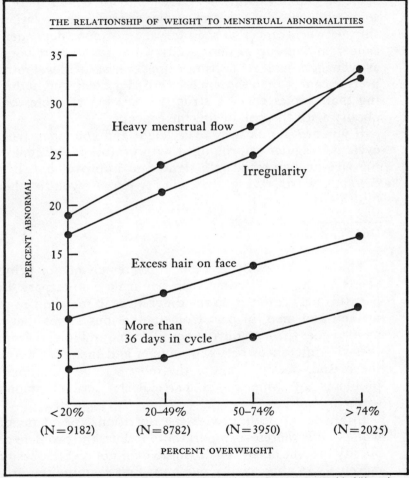

THE RELATIONSHIP OF WEIGHT TO MENSTRUAL ABNORMALITIES

argued that an increased amount of body fat will change a woman's hormonal balance and that the latter is what causes the abnormalities—a viewpoint for which there is some evidence, since several studies have shown a relationship between cancer of the uterus, a hormone-dependent cancer, and obesity. In one study women who were obese as teenagers had a 1.62 times greater risk of developing uterine cancer than those who were of normal weight during their adolescence—a strong association of adolescent obesity with the risk of uterine cancer.

If you are significantly overweight and your menstrual cycle is irregular or prolonged with profuse bleeding, losing weight may result in a significant improvement. It is certainly worth trying, since obesity exposes you to other health risks as well.

OBESITY

The newborn baby girl has a greater chance of being obese during her lifetime than her male counterpart. In part this may result from the differences in metabolism of women and men, in part from the various stages that a woman goes through during her life cycle and in part from lifestyle differences between women and men. Whatever the reason, obesity—one of the most serious nutritional problems in America—is particularly serious among women.

In any book dealing with the nutritional problems of women, it is therefore important to discuss the problem of obesity in some detail. To do this, we cannot regard obesity merely as an abnormality; we must first examine the process of weight control itself. An understanding of how the body maintains a given weight will help our understanding of how obesity may occur and how we may best prevent and treat it.

WEIGHT CONTROL

One of the great mysteries of nature is how the body is able to regulate its weight over long periods of time. There is no doubt that the factors that regulate the body's energy intake somehow communicate with those that regulate its energy output; it is well known that appetite increases with activity. In fact, the athlete may consume twice as much food as the sedentary individual. Conversely, if the amount of food is restricted, the body's physical activity will be markedly reduced. One of the body's first responses to starvation is a drastic curtailment of all nonessential physical activity, as if it were trying to maintain some hypothetical weight level by constantly adjusting its energy input and output.

Whatever the nature of the body's energy input-output communication system, it is certain that messages constantly pass between centers in the brain that regulate food intake and others that regulate energy expenditure. Some of these brain centers have actually been located, and their destruction in experimental animals has caused drastic abnormalities in appetite and energy regulation. For example, the brain center known as the hypothalamus contains a section that regulates appetite, and whose destruction results in uncontrolled eating. On the other hand, the destruction of another part of the hypothalamus results in a total loss of appetite. Centers that exert much finer degrees of control over the appetite must also exist, but have not yet been located. Despite this, research has recently begun to identify some of the reasons why some people maintain an almost constant weight no matter how much they eat or how active they are, whereas others constantly struggle to keep from gaining or losing a few pounds.

A person's weight depends not only on the amount of

food energy she or he consumes, but also on how efficiently that food energy is converted into heat for maintaining the body temperature and work energy for fueling the body's voluntary and automatic activities, for example, heartbeat and breathing. Let us examine two hypothetical persons. Both consume 2,500 calories per day in their diets. However, the body of one requires only 2,000 calories to maintain its normal temperature and perform all its necessary voluntary and automatic work, while the body of the other requires all 2,500 calories to fuel these processes. The result is that this second, more efficient body has 500 calories left over after expending the same amount of energy to maintain the same amount of activity. These 500 calories are then stored as body fat, presumably for use if food becomes scarce. From the standpoint of the chronic food shortages that plagued mankind for millions of years, the individual with the more efficient body would have the greater chance of survival, and we would expect nature to have favored such individuals and that they would today constitute a large percentage of the world's population.

But observe what happens when food becomes extremely abundant. Under such circumstances the more efficient individual begins to gain weight and deposit body fat at a greater rate than the less efficient individual; the price for efficiency in converting food calories into useful energy becomes obesity, which if carried to extremes will shorten the life expectancy of the energy-efficient individual and presumably, in the next million years, will increase the number of energy-inefficient individuals in the population.

In this sense, many obese persons "suffer" from having a particular type of metabolism which in a less food-abundant society would serve them well. In our society of abundance, however, they must maintain a lower food intake than average.

Studies in both Great Britain and the United States have begun to shed new light on the problem of energy use and obesity. In these studies, formerly obese persons who have been reduced to their ideal weights are put in a special environment in which their food intake is carefully controlled, all of their activities are carefully monitored and the energy required for these activities is calculated. It has been found that such formerly obese persons begin to gain weight at a calorie intake that is lower than that of persons who have been thin all their lives, even though both types begin the experiment at the same weight and expend the same amount of energy in the experiment. Thus, of two persons who weigh 150 pounds and get the same food, perform the same activities and expend the same energy, the one who always weighed 150 pounds will remain at that weight while the one who reduced to 150 pounds will begin to gain weight even though 150 pounds is his or her "ideal" weight. This ability to gain weight on fewer calories may be the most important reason for obesity in many people. Only by eating less than their thinner counterparts, by exercising more, or both can they hope to lose weight and keep it off over a long time.

The problem of constant calorie control to maintain one's ideal weight is much more prevalent in women than in men for two reasons: first because women often set their weight goal lower than what is ideal for them, with the result that their bodies rebel, struggling to maintain their lower weight; and second because women are more efficient calorie converters than men. But while this means that women survive longer than men and can utilize the limited calories available more efficiently during periods of food scarcity, it also means that they will begin to accumulate surplus calories sooner than men during periods of abundance, and will consequently deposit fat at a relatively smaller calorie intake.

For women, then, weight control is a double problem. Many are obese, while even greater numbers are too thin because of what they perceive as society's "ideal" weight for them. Such thinness may not be sufficient to threaten these women's health or longevity, but it may be enough to cause a constant "war" with their normal metabolism as a result of constantly having to diet. In fact at any given time, more than half of all women in America are on diets, many because they are truly too fat but many more because they wish to become or remain thin, and perhaps the majority suffer from a combination of these two problems.

TRUE OBESITY

While the definition of obesity as an excess amount of body fat may sound simple, it really is not. Excess can be defined only with precise standards that define the normal amount of fat in the human body at any stage of its development. Even the standards currently in use for normal body weights are, at best, approximations.

One reason why appropriate standards for body weight are difficult to establish is that we are interested in an individual's ideal weight—the weight at which that individual has the best chance to live longest and maintain optimal health—whereas health itself depends upon a host of factors. Added to this is the problem of measuring body fat, which requires complicated procedures and therefore cannot be done on large populations. The most common method for estimating body fat involves comparing an individual's weight with the average weight of persons of his or her height. This method has obvious drawbacks, since the 250-pound lineman on a professional football team may be heavy but is certainly not obese because most of his weight consists of muscle. One major task of science, then, is to determine an ideal weight-for-height range for men and women, and to decide how much extra weight above this range constitutes obesity.

A group that has traditionally used ideal weight-for-height curves has been the life insurance companies, which rely upon the curves to determine the weights at which people live longest. However, this too has some serious flaws, since the curves are likely to be based only on those people who seek life insurance. Moreover, small groups of people within the overweight population may contribute much more to the risk of dying prematurely than others. Obese people who come from families in which there has been a history of heart disease, for example, may influence a weight-for-height curve in such a way as to suggest that persons of similar weight without such a history may also have the risk of dying at a relatively early age. Another point is that the life-insurance curves use longevity as their sole basis; nothing relating to other aspects of health is considered. Finally, the curves now in use are more than twenty years old, whereas we know that today a person 5 to 10 percent heavier than the ideal weight on the 1959 life insurance charts actually has a better chance of achieving his or her maximum longevity. Currently, the life insurance tables are being modified to reflect this increase.

Notwithstanding all of the difficulties outlined above, we have learned a great deal in the last few decades about the health risks of obesity. For instance, we know that for most people, excess weight and excess fat are strongly associated, and that people who are 20 percent or more above their ideal weight have an increased risk of contracting several serious diseases. Furthermore, the risk of developing any of these diseases increases in direct proportion to the degree of obesity. Below is a list of a number of the diseases in which obesity is a direct causal factor, and some others that are strongly associated with obesity.

TABLE 1 DESIRABLE WEIGHTS FOR MEN AND WOMEN
AGED 25 AND OVER*

(in pounds according to height and frame, in indoor clothing)

	HEIGHT†	SMALL FRAME	MEDIUM FRAME	LARGE FRAME
		MEN		
Feet	Inches			
5	2	112–120	118–129	126–141
5	3	115–123	121–133	129–144
5	4	118–126	124–136	132–148
5	5	121–129	127–139	135–152
5	6	124–133	130–143	138–156
5	7	128–137	134–147	142–161
5	8	132–141	138–152	147–166
5	9	136–145	142–156	151–170
5	10	140–150	146–160	155–174
5	11	144–154	150–165	159–179
6	0	148–158	154–170	164–184
6	1	152–162	158–175	168–189
6	2	156–167	162–180	173–194
6	3	160–171	167–185	178–199
6	4	164–175	172–190	182–204
		WOMEN		
4	10	92–98	96–107	104–119
4	11	94–101	98–110	106–122
5	0	96–104	101–113	109–125
5	1	99–107	104–116	112–128
5	2	102–110	107–119	115–131
5	3	105–113	110–122	118–134
5	4	108–116	113–126	121–138
5	5	111–119	116–130	125–142
5	6	114–123	120–135	129–146
5	7	118–127	124–139	133–150
5	8	122–131	128–143	137–154
5	9	126–135	132–147	141–158
5	10	130–140	136–151	145–163
5	11	134–144	140–155	149–168
6	0	138–148	144–159	153–173

*Prepared by Metropolitan Life Insurance Co.; data derived primarily from Build and Blood
Pressure Study, 1959, Society of Actuaries.
†Height in shoes.

CAUSAL

PRIMARY CONTRIBUTING FACTOR
Diabetes
Menstrual abnormalities
Reproductive problems
Heart failure
Arthritis
Gout
High blood pressure

SECONDARY CONTRIBUTING FACTOR
Cancer of the uterus

ASSOCIATION
Atherosclerosis
Gall bladder disease
Premature death

Men who are overweight run a higher risk than over-weight women of developing some of these diseases, such as gout. For others, such as menstrual abnormalities or cancer of the uterus, women are exclusively at risk. For most, however, overweight members of both sexes bear an increased risk, with the net result that since more women than men are obese, obesity presents a greater health risk among women.

Clearly, then, women who are significantly overweight should try to lose weight, since obesity, like heavy cigarette smoking and heavy drinking, is a form of "Russian Roulette."

On the other hand, there is another aspect of obesity as a health risk. Suppose, for example, that a woman of a particular age, height and family background has a 20 percent chance of developing high blood pressure when she is at her ideal weight and a 40 percent chance if she is 25 percent over her ideal weight. The weight difference would double her risk of developing high blood pressure. However, more than half (60 percent) of overweight women with the same background as our hypothetical woman will not have high blood pressure. Thus, while it can be argued that since there are no known benefits of being overweight, all overweight persons should lose weight, the dilemma of which obese persons are at risk and which are not still constitutes a problem for medical science. If we could accurately identify those obese people with a high risk of developing a serious health problem, we would be able to counsel them with some assurance that our counsel would be of benefit.

At present, our ability to do this is limited. If, for example, you are overweight and your blood sugar tends to be above normal, health scientists can predict with some certainty that you stand a high chance of developing diabetes, and that this risk can be considerably reduced if you lose weight. But practically speaking, the ability to predict a health risk only after certain warning signals have already appeared means that overweight persons should pay particular attention to these signals and should see a physician more often than persons of average weight. As a general rule, an overweight person—particularly one over the age of forty—should have his or her blood pressure checked frequently and blood sugar and cholesterol tests at least once a year.

Obesity presents thorny problems in other respects as well. First, there is some evidence that overweight persons who do not develop any of the diseases listed above live slightly longer than their nonobese counterparts. For such people, losing weight may actually shorten their life expectancy. Second, most obese people have great difficulty reaching and maintaining their ideal weight, with the result that a significant portion of the overweight population will remain so until medical science learns how to deal more effectively with this problem.

One thing that is known is that it is much more difficult

to achieve permanent weight reduction if there are too many fat cells than if the fat cells are simply too full of fat. This is because, as discussed earlier in the book, the number of fat cells, once attained, cannot be reduced, whereas the amount of fat in each cell is very sensitive to the body's energy requirements.

Because the number of fat cells in the body is determined during childhood and adolescence, with the number of fat cells increasing very little, if at all in the adult, obesity can be separated into two types, one beginning in childhood or adolescence and characterized by too many fat cells, and the second beginning in adulthood (often in the so-called middle years) and characterized by a normal number of fat cells which are very swollen with excess fat.

At present we do not know whether one of these two types of obesity results in greater health risks than the other, although there are some indications—as we have already noted—that for certain diseases such as cancer of the uterus, too many fat cells may present a greater risk.

LOSING WEIGHT

In our discussion of energy efficiency, we have seen that weight reduction may be particularly difficult for the obese person not because of any lack of motivation but because of mechanisms within the body that favor the deposition of fat. From a practical standpoint this means that in order to lose weight, many obese people will have to reduce their caloric intake significantly.

Thus, while the first principle of weight reduction is reducing one's caloric intake, the extent of this reduction will vary from one overweight person to another. In extreme cases a diet providing 1,000 calories per day or less may be necessary, which can present a potentially serious problem since it is difficult for any diet of 1,500 calories or less to provide the daily requirements of all the known vitamins and minerals, much less for other essential nutrients whose requirements have not yet been determined. In fact, if a diet of less than 1,200 calories per day is needed to achieve weight loss, a vitamin and mineral supplement should be taken. Here again, then, is the need for a diet of high nutrient density, containing large quantities of essential nutrients per calorie. And since to meet these requirements the diet should be as varied as possible, the second principle of weight reduction is dietary variety.

The third principle of weight reduction is patience. It may be exciting to see the pounds come off rapidly, and there is often better motivation to continue a diet under such circumstances, but this may be neither practical nor safe for many obese people. Remember, as long as any weight loss is occurring the diet is working. Finally, it is important to increase one's energy expenditure while limiting one's calories. This will increase the negative energy balance and therefore the rate of weight loss. However, exercise alone without calorie control will usually not work, particularly in obese people, since even with vigorous exercise enough calories cannot be expended.

REDUCING CALORIC INTAKE

As we have seen, there are three ways in which your body can use up excess fat. The first is to consume fewer calories than your body needs for its conversion of food energy to metabolic energy. The second is to increase your caloric expenditure through voluntary activity, including exercise. Table 3 in Chapter 3 lists the caloric expenditure of many common forms of exercise. However, while exercise will "burn up" calories, it does not burn as many as you might think. Hence, exercise alone usually will not result in significant weight loss. Moreover, it will almost always lead to an increased appetite. Therefore some type of calorie control will have to be undertaken even with an exercise program. The third way in which to remove excess fat is to make your body less efficient in its use of calories, so that it uses more of the calories consumed in the diet for its energy needs. At present we do not have any safe method for decreasing the body's efficiency in converting food energy to metabolic energy. Certain drugs, particularly amphetamines, may do this, but are dangerous because they have side effects and put stress on the cardiovascular system, which can be particularly life-threatening in obese persons. Furthermore, after a short time the body develops a resistance to these drugs and they lose their efficacy. Certain diseases also make the body's conversion of food to energy less efficient. Perhaps the most dramatic example of this is cancer, which causes progressive weight loss despite what should be an adequate dietary intake. We do not understand how such disease states change the efficiency of conversion of the body's food intake to energy, but research is actively underway in this area.

Thus the only safe and effective way to induce your body to burn its own fat is to reduce your intake of calories to a level low enough to make your body use its own reserves —chiefly in the form of fat—to meet its energy needs.

Variety The importance of variety in a reducing diet has nothing to do with the ability of that diet to produce a weight loss; you will lose the same amount of weight if you take in 500 calories per day entirely from pineapples as you will if you consume the same 500 calories from a combination of different foods. Rather, variety is important in ensuring the safety of the diet, since any diet that restricts calories restricts essential nutrients, and if this restriction is severe enough or long enough, deficiencies of vitamins, minerals and even protein or essential fatty acids can occur.

Thus, the more strict a diet is or the longer it lasts, the more important variety becomes. For this reason it makes sense to begin with a diet that is both low in calories and rich in other nutrients. There are many ways of putting together such a diet, and some diets currently in use employ this principle of flexibility. A very effective diet is the one used by the New York City Health Department (and available to you free by writing to them), which is low in calories and provides a wide variety of foods with substitution options that allow the maximum in dietary flexibility. If the reducing diet you use limits your calories to levels below 1,000 for any length of time (more than a week), remember also to take a vitamin or mineral supplement; this should not substitute for variety in your food choices, but it will ensure that you get adequate amounts of these essential nutrients. If you are consuming fewer than 1,200 calories per day, an iron supplement becomes particularly important. For example, to construct a weight-reducing diet that would also meet the body's iron requirements, the architects of the Weight Watchers diet—an excellent calorie-restricted (1,200 calories) and well-balanced diet—had to include liver at least once a week. Unfortunately, many women will not eat liver and hence, even with a substitute, will fall short of their iron requirement unless they take a fortified substitute such as cereals.

Patience Not all overweight persons will lose weight at the same rate. No diet can assure you that within the first week or two of dieting you will lose five or ten pounds. We have seen that the body has ways of balancing its food intake and energy output to keep its weight relatively constant, and it is very important to remember that it is continuously adjusting its metabolism to "defend" or maintain a particular weight even while you diet. Even if you overwhelm these defenses by reducing your caloric intake to very low levels your weight loss may be slow. Therefore patience is an important part of any reducing diet.

Actually there is an advantage to losing weight over a long period of time: it gives the body time to "retrain" itself to defend a lower weight. And don't be fooled: an initial rapid weight loss on any reducing diet means that you are losing water, not fat. This is a temporary state that your body goes through as it adjusts to your new eating pattern. Thus, while it may be reassuring to see those pounds drop off quickly as you begin a new diet, remember that this initial rapid loss is likely to be followed by a "leveling off" period. When this happens, do not be disheartened. You are still losing weight, or at least body fat, even though the scale may not show it. What is actually happening is that you are reaccumulating some of the water you lost initially, while at the same time burning off some of your stored fat. As soon as your body has rehydrated itself, you will again experience a measurable weight loss. After this, as long as your weight continues to decrease, even if only by a half pound per week, keep at it until you reach your desirable weight.

You may feel frustrated by the slowness of your weight loss, but by giving your body the chance to readjust you may prevent the most frustrating of all dieting experiences: regaining all of your lost weight after the diet is over.

MAINTAINING A REDUCED WEIGHT

Weight maintenance after successful weight loss is much more difficult than losing weight initially. Part of the difficulty stems from unreasonable goals. From what we have seen, an obese woman may have a much harder time maintaining her ideal weight than a lean woman simply because of her more efficient conversion of food energy to metabolic energy. This is particularly true for the woman who has been obese since childhood because she has too many fat cells. By the same token, many obese women gain weight more readily than their lean counterparts. The key here is compromise—setting a long-term goal that may not be ideal but that is achievable. This may mean eating less food or consuming fewer calories than before, but at a reasonably reduced level. Often, success will require a change in lifestyle or at least in one's overall eating pattern —which is one reason why behavior modification techniques have worked so well with overweight persons.

Similarly, there is no reason for rigidity in a reducing diet or weight-maintenance plan. The reduced number of daily calories for either of these need not be kept at the same level each day. In fact, no living creature normally takes in the same number of calories daily. Instead, successful weight loss and maintenance, both psychologically and physically, depend upon changing one's overall pattern of food consumption over a long period without setting daily caloric goals.

CANCER OF THE BREAST

No disease is more feared by women than cancer of the breast. As with most cancers, the exact cause of breast cancer remains unknown. Currently, most experts believe that as many as 60 percent of all cancers are somehow related to the environment in which we live, including the food we consume. In fact, there have been many claims about how nutrition may be related to breast cancer. Most of these cannot be substantiated; however, solid scientific evidence has recently related one component of the diet to the incidence of breast cancer. That component is fat.

Because it is important for all women to understand the evidence upon which this conclusion is based, I will review this evidence briefly. But even more important is to decide what to do in the face of the evidence. Here, even though we do not know all the answers, we can at least tentatively make certain recommendations. Finally, we can help to dispel some nutritional myths about breast cancer.

Scientists routinely induce cancer in animals by injecting them with chemicals known as carcinogens. Furthermore, different types of carcinogens induce different types of cancers, and some cause cancer of the breast in mice. During the course of experiments such as these it was noted that certain carcinogens caused cancer of the breast in large numbers of mice only if the animals were being maintained on a relatively high fat diet. When these experiments were continued, a direct and measurable relationship was found between the amount of fat in the diet and the ability of various carcinogens to induce breast cancer: the higher the total fat content of the diet the greater was the incidence of such cancer. No reason has yet been revealed for this, but further experiments have uncovered subtle differences in the types and amounts of hormones produced by animals raised on high- and low-fat diets. Because these hormones are involved in breast development and function, it has been postulated that changes in the hormones alter conditions within the breast, making it more susceptible to the effects of carcinogens.

A number of different types of studies with women support the data collected from the animal experiments. The most compelling evidence comes from the observation that in populations of women where fat consumption is low, the incidence of breast cancer is low, while the opposite is true in populations where there is a high consumption of fat. Figure 3 relates the incidence of breast cancer to fat consumption in different countries throughout the world.

Note that in Denmark and New Zealand, where fat consumption is high, the incidence of breast cancer is high. By

FIGURE 3

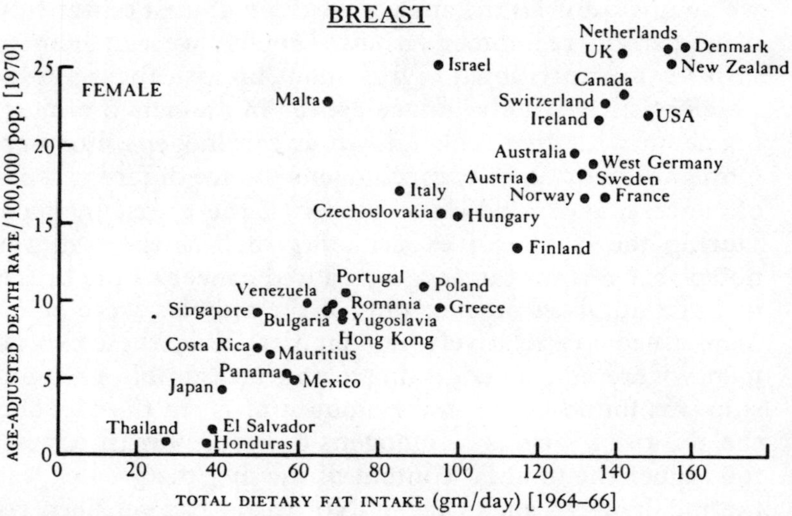

BREAST

Correlation between per capita consumption of dietary fat (25) and age-adjusted mortality from breast cancer in different countries (2). Mortality for the United States was estimated from values given for U.S. white and U.S. nonwhite, and that for the United Kingdom from values given for England and Wales, Scotland, and Northern Ireland. Although not specified in the latest compilation, earlier data on the death rate from breast cancer in Israel was based on the Jewish population only, and this may account for its failure to conform to the correlation with fat intake. The data from Malta should probably be investigated more thoroughly to see whether there is a rational explanation for its failure to conform.

From: K. K. Carroll, Dietary Factors in Hormone-Dependent Cancers in Nutrition and Cancer, *ed. M. Winick,* (New York: John Wiley & Sons, 1977), p. 28.

contrast, in Thailand and Honduras, where fat consumption is low, the incidence of breast cancer is low. In the United States the consumption of dietary fat is relatively high and the incidence of breast cancer is likewise relatively high.

Other types of studies have strengthened this evidence of a link between dietary fat consumption and the incidence of breast cancer, and have further suggested that a high dietary fat intake may be important not only in mid- and later life, when breast cancer most often occurs, but much earlier in life, since breast cancer as well as other cancers may take many years to appear. Still other studies, on the incidence of breast cancer in populations in both their country of origin where fat intake is low and after migration to a new country where the fat intake is high have further confirmed the fat/breast-cancer correlation. In Japan, for instance, fat intake is low and breast cancer rates are also low, and Japanese women who migrate to the United States usually maintain the rate of breast cancer seen in Japan. It is unclear whether this is because they continue to eat a Japanese diet or whether they have not been exposed to the high-fat Western diet for long enough. Their daughters, however, show a markedly different pattern, being afflicted with breast cancer in the same numbers as American women, in conjunction with the American diet. Similar studies with European Jews who have migrated to Israel suggest the same outcome.

The evidence that a high-fat diet is in some way related to breast cancer is therefore very strong. What remains unknown in humans is precisely *how* a high-fat diet increases the risk of breast cancer. Does it work as in animals, by increasing one's susceptibility to the effects of carcinogens in the environment? Or does it work more directly, through the fat itself or some component of the fat? Although scientists suspect that the first explanation is the more probable, the second possibility cannot be ruled out. Therefore, research is proceeding in both directions. Whichever explanation proves to be correct (and perhaps both are), the best way to lower your risk for breast cancer is to lower your total fat intake. This, then, is an important reason to follow the advice of the American Heart Association, the National Academy of Science and the Departments of Health and Human Services and of Agriculture: Reduce the fat in your diet to 30 percent of your caloric intake.

The nature of the fat you consume appears to be less important in the case of breast cancer than in atherosclerosis (hardening of the arteries) and heart disease. In animals, high amounts of either saturated or unsaturated fat increase the rate at which experimentally produced breast cancer develops. In humans the correlation is much stronger with the total fat intake than with the amount of saturated or unsaturated fat in the diet. Therefore, at least with regard to breast cancer, polyunsaturated fats and cooking oils would not appear to make a difference in the risk, and they do count toward the 30 percent fat total in the daily caloric intake. Within this 30 percent it is all right to increase the ratio of polyunsaturated fat.

Recently scientists have begun to find another relationship between certain cancers and diet. In populations whose diets have a low vitamin A content, the incidence of various cancers is somewhat higher. Although this link has not been firmly established for breast cancer, there are certain reasons why it may be exist. Although the evidence is still far from complete, this is a good reason for maintaining an adequate vitamin A intake in your diet, and an impetus to eat foods that are high in vitamin A (primarily yellow vegetables, certain meats and fish). On the other hand, simply because a deficiency of vitamin A may be bad, do not assume that an excess is good. Unfortunately, even though the data linking vitamin A to the possible risk of cancer are inconclusive they are already being misinterpreted, with some people advocating long-term supplementation with high doses of vitamin A to protect against many cancers including cancer of the breast. High doses of vitamin A for long periods can be very dangerous, and should not be taken, especially since there is no evidence that they offer any more cancer protection than a good diet. By the same token, there is no evidence to support claims that vitamin E and vitamin C in large doses will prevent breast cancer.

In fact, more myths may surround the subject of nutrition and breast cancer than any other aspect of nutrition. Perhaps the most destructive of these is that breast feeding your infant will increase your chances for developing breast cancer—a claim for which there is absolutely no truth whatsoever. Definitive studies have shown no difference in the incidence of breast cancer among women who breast feed and those who do not, and a study in Hong Kong, where women traditionally feed their infants from only one breast, has shown a higher incidence of breast cancer in the unnursed breast. This does not necessarily suggest that women who do not breast feed at all have a greater risk of developing breast cancer than those who do, but it certainly reinforces the concept that breast feeding is absolutely safe from the standpoint of breast-cancer risk.

MENOPAUSE

A woman's ability to have babies comes to an end with menopause. At some time around the age of fifty the ovaries stop producing mature eggs and the secretion of reproductive hormones, especially estrogen, decreases markedly. These changes alter the pattern of menstruation and often create unpleasant symptoms. These often include flushing (hot flashes), headache, dizziness, nervousness and digestive abnormalities. Many women also complain of muscle and joint pain and of a constant feeling of tiredness. Finally, in about one-third of women menopause is accompanied by weight gain and obesity.

The alteration in the menstrual pattern that occurs with menopause varies from one woman to another. In some there is a gradual lessening of the menstrual blood flow without any irregularities. In others, the menstrual periods will be relatively normal but some will be missed. In still others both the menstrual rhythm and the amount of menstrual flow will be affected. Finally, in some women menstruation will cease abruptly with menopause. Whatever the pattern, the end result is the same: menstruation ceases and the ability to conceive and bear children is lost. However, this is the only aspect of a woman's life that is lost. Women are just as capable of fulfilling and enjoying every other personal, familial, and vocational aspect of life after menopause as they were before. In fact many women report more enjoyment of sex after menopause than before it because of the disappearance of fear of accidental conception.

From the standpoint of nutrition, both the physiological changes and the accompanying symptoms that occur during menopause are extremely important. The cessation of menstrual flow means an end to the loss of large quantities of iron every month, and the dietary iron requirement drops sharply. Nor with the end of bleeding is there any longer a need for the formation of large numbers of new blood cells, and the requirements for zinc and folic acid therefore also decrease.

Thus, the physiological changes of menopause generally reduce the need for certain key nutrients. However, another physiologic change occurs at menopause which increases the need for one nutrient, calcium. Because of the hormonal changes that occur at this time, the body loses calcium much more rapidly than it did before.

It is unclear whether the obesity that frequently occurs at menopause results directly from the hormonal changes that take place at this time or whether it is secondary to the "mood" changes during menopause. Whatever the cause may be, the result is the same: one-third of all women who go through menopause gain too much weight. To prevent this from happening, reduce your calorie intake by consuming a wide variety of nutrient-dense foods and stay active, at least as active as you were before.

However, beyond the general need to avoid gaining weight during menopause the symptoms that accompany this period of change impose their own special nutritional problems. The hot flashes of menopause are thought to result from the instability of the smaller blood vessels, which alternately expand (causing the hot flashes) or contract (causing sweating or chilliness and pallor). The changes in body temperature that occur during these periods of flushing and chilliness, if they last for any length of time, alter the body's calorie requirement. Even more important is that these changes, with the symptoms of headache, dizziness and nervous anxiety that may also occur, can lead to erratic eating patterns. In response to such discomforts, a woman will sometimes increase her consumption of high-calorie foods, contributing to the already present danger of obesity. Alternatively, some women lose their appetites, creating the risk of nutrient deficiencies.

Following the nutritional guidelines we have discussed throughout this book—including the use of a varied, high-nutrient-density diet, an adequate intake of the essential vitamins and minerals, and regular exercise—is the answer to many of the nutritional difficulties of menopause. Yet unfortunately, because this period is one of great concern to women, many fall prey to all sorts of schemes promising to delay or prevent menopause, and in some cases to reverse the changes that have already occurred. Don't be fooled: no vitamin or mineral in any dose will delay menopause or bring back menstruation. Instead, concentrate on eating calcium-rich foods, taking supplements if necessary. If your food preferences or a lack of appetite interfere with the dietary approach to this, a calcium supplement of 500 milligrams per day will help to meet your needs. And keep active; activity minimizes calcium loss from the bones and uses up calories that might otherwise be converted to fat. Finally, watch your weight. If it begins to climb, cut your calories.

Beyond these two primary concerns, calcium and calories, remember that after menopause, you have fifteen or twenty more years before the special nutritional stresses of aging begin to occur—twenty years of active, productive life with few of the nutritional concerns of your younger days. Build up your iron and zinc reserves. You will need them later on. The same is true, although to a lesser extent, for your vitamin B_{12} intake. Avoid obesity; at this time of life it is a particular health risk. We have outlined how you can accomplish these goals. The time between menopause and old age is the easiest time to do it.

CHAPTER 8

The Mature Years

One of the most important aspects of any discussion of the postreproductive years is the distinction between longevity and the process of aging. Certainly the two are related. As one adds more years of life she or he undergoes a series of changes that constitute the aging process. But the process of aging is not built only around the calendar; to a much greater extent it depends upon a biological schedule that proceeds at a different rate in different people. We have all seen "young" eighty-year-olds and "old" fifty-year-olds. And this does not apply to appearance only; the biology of the body, indeed its whole metabolism and physiology, may reflect aging in a young person and relative youth in an old one.

The distinction between longevity and aging is particularly important for women. In our society, women live almost ten years longer than men. At least in part, this seems to be because of an inherent difference between males and females, for among almost all mammals the female of the species lives longer than the male. For example, men's arteries appear to age more quickly than women's. This will lead to earlier heart disease, stroke and kidney problems. On the other hand, in some ways women age faster than men, such as in the loss of calcium from their bones. Thus, although it is obviously important to all of us to live as long as we can, it is equally important to slow down the rate at which we age so that we can make the most of our lifespan. Proper nutrition can play a role in both processes, and can specifically affect the rate of aging in women.

In the following sections we will address the nutritional considerations that are important in extending one's lifespan, and the nutritional aspects of this that specifically concern women. Yet no matter how good our nutrition may be, we must all age, and as the human lifespan increases with progress in science and medicine we will spend more years with our bodies both physically and chronologically older. Therefore, we must also direct our attention to the older body, with its older organs, which requires different quantities of nutrients than in youth and the middle years. And once again, the nature of these differences in nutritional requirements is different in women and men. If these adjusted quantities are supplied the body will function efficiently. If not, distress and even disease may ensue.

LONGEVITY

You have undoubtedly heard—and probably from many sources—that high doses of certain vitamins or minerals taken every day will increase your lifespan. Vitamins C, E and A are currently enjoying popularity as "life extenders." Among the minerals, calcium and more recently selenium have been heralded as prolonging life. Most of these claims are based on no data at all. Some are outright misinterpretations or unwarranted projections based on studies with animals.

This is not to say that certain nutritional practices will not favor an increased lifespan. Obese persons who lose weight can expect to add to their longevity. To the extent that reducing dietary fat reduces the incidence of fatal heart attacks and also that it reduces the risk of some types of cancer it will extend life. Moreover, although we have not learned of any specific nutritional pattern that is guaranteed to increase life expectancy, we have learned, primarily from animal experiments, that certain nutritional patterns even very early in life may be important in determining longevity. Rats fed a reduced calorie diet during the pre- and post-weaning periods, for instance, live longer than those given a high-calorie diet. Such data may not be directly relevant to humans, but if you want to increase your chances for a long life it certainly makes more sense to control your weight throughout your younger years than to pop vitamin and mineral supplements throughout your middle and older years. Such supplements certainly have their proper place in nutrition, but their use in this manner detracts from the real and sometimes more difficult nutritional habits that have been demonstrated to increase longevity, and also creates a false sense of security, since those who advocate vitamin and mineral tablets as a means for prolonging life are perpetrating a cruel hoax.

If you truly wish to increase your chances for a long life, some sound recommendations for how to do this are given below. These recommendations are not new. They have been made by the American Heart Association and by the Departments of Health and Human Services and of Agriculture; and recently, in relation to cancer, they have been made by a committee of the National Academy of Sciences. And while implementing this kind of dietary pattern may be more difficult than taking a vitamin-mineral supplement each morning, it can be done by most people without a major change in lifestyle. More important is that, while these dietary changes cannot guarantee you another five or ten years of life, they increase your chances of living longer by decreasing your risk of developing certain fatal diseases.

Keep your weight as close to ideal as possible; both overweight and underweight are associated with a reduced life expectancy. This problem is particularly relevant to women, since both obesity and underweight are more prevalent among women. If you eat the typical American diet, reduce your intake of total and saturated fat. This will reduce your chances of suffering a heart attack and, particularly with regard to women, may reduce your chances for developing breast cancer.

Reduce your intake of salt. This will reduce your risk of developing high blood pressure and your chances of developing heart disease or having a stroke.

Increase your consumption of dietary fiber (found mostly in unrefined foods). This may decrease your risk of developing certain cancers of the gastrointestinal tract.

DELAYING THE AGING PROCESS

For women, perhaps the most serious consequence of aging is a progressive decalcification of the bones that results in pain and disability and may end in fractures of those bones that bear most of the weight of the body. When severe, this process is termed osteoporosis. It is much more common among women than among men because it proceeds more rapidly in women.

There are several important reasons for this difference between the sexes. First, women begin to lose calcium from their bones at an earlier age than men. By the third decade of life many women are already in what is known as a negative calcium balance, in which they are losing more calcium than they are getting into their bodies. Second, men have bigger and wider bones and hence have greater calcium stores than women. Third, as we have seen, women during certain stages of their life cycle—especially pregnancy and lactation—have markedly increased demands for calcium. Fourth, there is an abrupt change during menopause in a woman's hormonal status, which dramatically increases calcium loss from the bones.

We are just beginning to understand the reason for this rapid loss of calcium that begins in menopause and progresses through a woman's later years. Part of the problem is that the kidney loses some of its ability to convert vitamin D into the active form in which the vitamin promotes calcium absorption. Hence the most important stimulus to calcium absorption is decreased, and the body absorbs less calcium from the diet. There is also some evidence that the intestinal cells themselves cannot absorb and transport dietary calcium as well as they can in the years before menopause. Finally, since the loss of bone calcium is a progressive process, more calcium is lost as a person gets older, and because women live an average of about ten years longer than men, they can expect ten more years of bone demineralization at a relatively rapid rate.

Thus at any given age women will have less calcium in their bones than men, and as a result will—particularly after menopause—have more brittle bones than men. It is this that results in the higher incidence of fractured hips and fractured vertebrae in older women than in comparably aged men. In fact, since in the very senior years there are many more women than men, the total number of these fractures among women is ten times higher among women than among men.

What can a woman do to reduce her rate of calcium loss and minimize her risk for developing osteoporosis and its painful and debilitating consequences? A great deal, according to scientists' findings. And what is most important from our focus is that much of this can be accomplished by dietary means.

Before we can really understand the importance of nutrition in delaying the onset and slowing the progression of osteoporosis, we should take a brief look at how the body gains and loses calcium.

Ninety-nine percent of the body's calcium resides in our bones. Together with phosphorus, this calcium in bone forms a complex substance known as hydroxyapatite, which gives bone its hardness and structural integrity. The other 1 percent of the body's calcium is spread throughout every cell in the body. This 1 percent of calcium, even though a relatively small amount, is crucial for the proper functioning of all of the body's tissues and organs. Without it, brain cells cannot send impulses and muscle cells cannot contract. In actuality this 1 percent itself constitutes a greater absolute amount of calcium than the amount of many of the vital trace minerals in the body, including zinc, copper, magnesium and selenium. In fact, it is so important that the body has a specific mechanism for keeping the amount of this calcium at an appropriate level. One way in which the body does this is through the bones, which constantly supply calcium to the blood for transport to the cells, while at the same time removing calcium from the blood to maintain their own structural integrity. We call this a state of dynamic equilibrium—dynamic because calcium is constantly moving in one direction or another; equilibrium because a constant level of calcium is maintained in the non-skeletal tissues. If the concentration of

The Mature Years

calcium in the blood begins to fall, the bones release calcium into the blood to make up the deficit; if the calcium concentration in the blood gets too high, the bones extract the excess. Accordingly, we can view bone as a tissue in which calcium is constantly "turning over," with molecules of calcium constantly going in and out. It acts as a reservoir when the other tissues need more calcium and as a dam when they are getting too much.

But the body cannot manufacture calcium; it depends upon the diet as its major source of this essential mineral. Yet while many foods are rich in calcium—particularly the dairy foods and green leafy plant foods that we have already discussed—the amount of calcium that the body actually absorbs depends only partly on the amount of calcium in the foods we eat; a complex interaction of other nutrients and hormones exerts a major influence on the amount of calcium absorbed through the gastrointestinal tract into the blood. As we saw earlier, phosphorus, the other mineral that makes up the hydroxyapatite in the bones, is very important in this respect. With calcium, it is carried, by the same "carrier" protein, through the cells that line the intestine and into the blood; both minerals therefore ride on the same "train," and both compete for the same "seats." Every seat filled by a phosphorus particle is one less seat for a calcium particle. It is for this reason that consuming phosphorus in a calcium-containing meal limits the amount of calcium that will get into the body. And it is because of this that many dairy products may not be the most efficient foods from which to get our calcium, since they also have a high phosphorus content, as do meat and many carbonated soft drinks. It is interesting in this regard that breast milk, the infant's only source of calcium, contains much less phosphorus than cow's milk. Remember, a period of at least one hour should be left between ingestion of a calcium-containing food and the ingestion of a large portion of meat or a phosphate-containing soft drink to promote optimal calcium absorption. Thus a salad with cottage cheese is a much better source of calcium than a steak with baked potato and sour cream, even though the cottage cheese and the sour cream may contain roughly the same amount of calcium. By the same token, a dish of ice cream following a pizza or a spaghetti dinner will supply more usable calcium than it could after a hamburger or roast beef sandwich. And although an ice cream soda may be delicious and even lower in fat and calories a malted milk will supply more calcium.

Table 1 lists a number of foods that provide 300 mg of calcium per serving, or about one-third the total daily requirement. The nondairy sources will be absorbed somewhat better than the dairy sources because of their lower phosphorus content, but all of these foods are excellent sources of calcium and one or more portions per day of any one of them will get you well on your way to meeting your calcium requirements.

By far the most important nutrient controlling the absorption of calcium is vitamin D. In fact, the principal role of this vitamin is to facilitate calcium absorption. In our discussion of pregnancy and the placenta, we saw how, in order to make this hormone, the kidney must convert dietary vitamin D into a slightly different compound which then acts on the cells of the gastrointestinal tract, causing these cells to take up more calcium and transfer it to the blood stream. Therefore, as a potent influence on dietary calcium absorption, vitamin D helps to prevent the resorption of calcium from the bones in order to keep the blood and tissue levels high.

A varied diet, particularly one rich in calcium, will provide more than enough vitamin D. Additionally, even moderate exposure to sunlight will permit the ultraviolet rays of the sun to activate the inactive form of the vitamin stored

TABLE 1   CALCIUM SOURCES
(Each portion provides approximately 300 mg calcium)

FOOD	WEIGHT	SERVING
Almonds, chopped	130 grams	1 cup
Buttermilk	245 grams	8 oz.
Cheddar cheese	42 grams	1½ oz.
Collard greens, chopped, cooked from frozen package	170 grams	1 cup
Cottage cheese, creamed or uncreamed	340 grams	12 oz.
Evaporated milk, unsweetened	126 grams	4 oz.
Fluid milk, whole or skim lowfat	245 grams	8 oz.
(with 2% milk solids added)	245 grams	7 oz.
Kale, cooked from frozen pkg.	260 grams	2 cups
Mackerel, Pacific, canned	100 grams	3½ oz.
Tofu (soybean curd)	240 grams	2 pieces
Turnip greens, cooked from froz. pkg.	165 grams	1½ cups
Raisins	165 grams	1 cup
Prunes, uncooked, without pits	154 grams	⅞ cup

in the skin, which can then be sent to the kidney for conversion into its active form. However, since the kidney will convert only as much of the vitamin as is needed to provide the tiny quantity of vitamin D hormone for promoting optimal calcium absorption, excess dietary or supplemental vitamin D will not be converted. Therefore, do not rely upon vitamin D supplements to provide your needs of this vital nutrient. They will not provide a kind of "insurance." Moreover, too much vitamin D can be toxic. So don't be fooled by slick advertisements advocating high doses of vitamin D to protect your bones! They are irresponsible and dangerous.

Several factors directly influence calcium loss from the bones. One of these is the amount of dietary protein. The higher the protein content of the diet the more calcium is lost from the bones.

The recommendation regarding total protein intake recognizes that too much of a good thing is not always desirable. An adequate amount of protein is absolutely essential for good health, but Americans generally consume far more protein than they need. Thus the word here is moderation—less meat and more grains, fruits and vegetables. This does not mean a vegetarian diet, although vegetarians are well off from the standpoint of calcium balance, but rather cutting down on the quantity of meat in your diet, particularly if you follow the typical American eating pattern.

Another important cause of calcium loss from the bones is prolonged inactivity, and particularly bed rest. During such periods, calcium loss from the bones is accelerated. Conversely, active exercise reduces this loss. An example of what happens with inactivity can be seen in astronauts. During a week's space flight, as much as 5 percent of their bodies' calcium may be lost from the bones. Unless rapidly corrected, this condition may result in long-term problems, such as osteoporosis, particularly in women astronauts.

There is no doubt that moderate amounts of exercise promote calcium deposition into the bones. Thus, the sooner you make regular exercise a part of your lifestyle the better. You don't have to overdo it; regular exercise is more important than the actual nature of the exercise itself. However, exercises that make your bones bear weight, such as walking, jogging, bicycle riding, and gymnastics, are particularly useful. If your bones are already weakened from calcium loss you should institute an exercise program very carefully, after consulting a physician and under proper supervision. This is especially true after a period of bed rest because of illness. Under such circumstances your bones will have lost calcium; with care, you will benefit immensely by replacing that calcium, through diet and exercise, after the illness is over.

From this brief description we can draw up a balance sheet with which most older women can minimize the net calcium loss from their bones. Although this approach may not completely reverse the negative calcium balance present in most older women, it should increase the time necessary for the development of osteoporosis. On the intake side are enough calcium in the diet; minimum amounts of phosphorus in calcium-containing meals; adequate amounts of vitamin D either in the diet or derived from exposing the skin to sunlight; and a kidney that is capable of converting this vitamin D into its active form. On the output side are the need to reduce the dietary protein intake and to exercise the muscles and joints with activities that promote weight bearing.

In fact, while the above recommendations are highly useful for older women, a woman should try to start following them as early in life as possible, and should continue to abide by them throughout her entire life; they are relevant at any age. If you promote this approach during infancy and early childhood, as new bone is being laid down, the amount of calcium that will be taken into the body will be very high because the kidney is very active in making the vitamin D hormone at this time. The bones will then not only mineralize properly but extra calcium will be stored for later use. During adolescence, as the bones again begin to grow, calcium absorption again becomes much more efficient, and the approach outlined above will again help to ensure that a generous amount of calcium is stored in the bones. If the same approach is used during pregnancy and lactation, when there are very heavy calcium demands placed on the mother, her body will also respond by absorbing calcium much more efficiently, meaning that she need not end a pregnancy or nursing period with significant amounts of calcium lost from her bones, and may in fact finish pregnancy and lactation with a net calcium gain. In the third decade of life, which is when most women go into a negative calcium balance, the same rules can sharply reduce the body's calcium loss and increase the amount of calcium held in reserve when menopause is reached.

NEWER DEVELOPMENTS IN THE TREATMENT OF OSTEOPOROSIS

In the last few years, medical science has made a major breakthrough that will hopefully offer relief for millions of women suffering from varying degrees of osteoporosis. With the discovery of the active vitamin D hormone that is made in the kidney, and the finding that the aging kidney loses its ability to produce this hormone, scientists began to question whether such decreased amounts of the hormone were in some way related to osteoporosis. When subsequent studies showed that levels of the hormone were particularly low in women with osteoporosis, efforts were undertaken to make the hormone artificially and use it to treat the condition. Within the last few years the hormone has been synthesized and is now available with a doctor's prescription. The few trials in which it has been used to treat severe osteoporosis have so far been very encouraging. The synthetic hormone has been found to increase calcium absorption, and calcium has actually been deposited in the bones of osteoporosis patients who have received it. Although it is too early to tell how useful this treatment will be, you should consult your physician about its use if you have osteoporosis; it must be used under strict medical supervision because it is very potent and when given in excess can be dangerous. Remember, ordinary vitamin D in large doses has no place in the treatment of osteoporosis.

CALCIUM AND PERIODONTAL DISEASE

Another effect of aging that is related to the depletion of calcium from the bones is periodontal disease, the major

cause of tooth loss in older people. About 20 percent of
Americans over seventy have lost all their teeth, a condition which in itself leads to nutritional problems. Periodontal disease does not have the high prevalence among
women that osteoporosis does. However, because it
becomes progressively more common with age, and because women constitute a larger proportion of the elderly
population, periodontal disease—like osteoporosis—does
ultimately affect many more women than men.

Periodontal disease can be described as a vicious cycle
with two major components: infection and bone loss. Den-
tists and other health professionals disagree to some extent
about which of these precedes the other. Most experts feel
that the disease begins with infection of the gums, which
in turn leads to erosion of the bony sockets in the jaw that
hold the roots of the teeth. As the sockets wear away, the
teeth loosen, aggravating the infection, which then further
erodes the bone. On the other hand, some experts feel that
the process begins in the same way as osteoporosis, with the
loss of calcium from the jaw bones. This leads to loosening
of the teeth and sore gums, which then become infected
and initiate the same cycle as above.

Regardless of the way in which periodontal disease begins, nutrition plays a role in its cause and under certain
circumstances in its treatment. In terms of treating the
bone erosion caused by calcium loss, the same nutritional
principles hold as for osteoporosis: a diet consisting of calcium-rich foods; a reduced phosphorus intake at calcium-
containing meals; a lower overall protein consumption;
and adequate amounts of vitamin D. From the standpoint
of the infection, good oral hygiene, including frequent
toothbrushing (which will reduce the numbers of infectious bacteria on the teeth and gums), is important. Additionally, some studies have suggested that *a limited number*
of people with periodontal disease may benefit from cal-

cium supplementation; in some cases it has reduced the need for extensive dental treatment of the disease and in a few has even eliminated this need. Thus, although the reasons for its effectiveness are not understood, such supplementation may prove worthwhile if you suffer from periodontal disease.

HIGH BLOOD PRESSURE

The blood pressure is the pressure that blood exerts on the walls of the arteries and veins through which it passes as it circulates around the body. Although a slow but steady increase in blood pressure was long considered part of the normal aging process, and a tendency to high blood pressure (hypertension) was therefore believed to be a natural accompaniment of aging, medical science has recently discovered that blood pressure increases with age only in populations that consume relatively large amounts of salt. Thus, only when salt—and more precisely sodium, which is the constituent of salt that affects the blood pressure—is consumed in large amounts can we expect older people to have high blood pressure. Therefore, rather than being a disease that is normally more common in elderly persons generally, hypertension is a disease that is more common among elderly persons who have consumed too much salt throughout their early and middle years. In countries in which the diet contains but small amounts of salt, the blood pressure does not increase with age.

Unfortunately, Americans consume too much salt, and older Americans therefore have higher blood pressures than younger ones. In fact, in countries such as the United States in which salt intake is moderately high, there is a direct correlation between blood pressure and age, with older populations having higher blood pressures. And because American women live longer than American men, more of them—as in the case of several other diseases—will suffer from hypertension.

Theoretically, then, a major way to reduce your risk of developing high blood pressure in your later years is to reduce your use of salt and sodium-containing foods at an earlier age. In practice, however, this is not always so easy. Obviously, reducing or stopping your use of the salt shaker will help. Using less salt during cooking will also help. But large amounts of salt and sodium are added to many of the foods we buy, and if we really want to limit our sodium intake we must be aware of this. Some brands of canned peas contain 100 times as much sodium as fresh peas. Therefore, read labels! Is sodium listed as an ingredient? If so, does the label say how much? Compare this with other similar products, and choose the one with the lowest sodium content. If salt is listed, but the amount is not given, see where it is placed among the ingredients. The higher it is on the list the more is being used. Some products do not list the quantity of sodium or salt on the label. If the general public, and especially women, who do most of the food buying for themselves and their families, shopped with "low sodium" in mind, the message to the food industry would be unmistakable. In fact, the message is beginning to get through, for when such products as salt-free potato chips are being offered you know the food industry is listening.

What is that? "Food without salt tastes bland. Taking salt away will destroy the enjoyment of eating"?

The preference for a salty taste in foods is a learned one. The more salt in the foods we eat the more salt is required to satisfy our taste buds. Infants are not born with a preference for salt; they learn by exposure. And since this preference has to be learned, losing it requires a period of retraining. Certainly the sudden elimination of most of the sodium in their diets will make eating a dull experience for many people. But slowly reducing one's salt intake over a period of months will often work. In fact many people have said that they did not know how good foods could taste until they stopped drowning them in salt. So begin by tasting your food before you add salt; then add progressively less and less with each passing week and month. Next, add less salt to the foods you cook. You don't have to eliminate it altogether, but you can cut back appreciably. Finally, use products that have a relatively low sodium content, and cut down on such highly salted foods as pickled meats, fish, and vegetables and cold cuts; you don't have to eliminate them completely from your diet; but use them only occasionally and in small amounts. Table 2 is a list of foods that are high in sodium.

TABLE 2	FOODS HIGH IN SODIUM

Buttermilk
Canned tuna fish
Many canned vegetables (read label)
All "pickled" foods
All smoked foods
Cold cuts
Sausages
Salted crackers and pretzels
Cheese and cheese spreads
Bouillon, dehydrated soups
Soy sauce, mustard, ketchup, commercial salad
   preparations and seasoning salts

For persons who already have hypertension the problem is quite different than for those who are seeking to avoid it. Here the gradual reduction of salt in the diet is not enough. In fact the only way to control the high blood pressure by dietary means alone is to drastically reduce your salt intake to very low levels. In our society, however, this is very difficult; it means eating only certain foods, all but eliminating processed foods from one's diet, and restricting meals away from home to a very few establishments that will cater to people on a very low salt diet. Because salt in the diet is practically unavoidable, most physicians treat hypertension with blood-pressure-reducing drugs combined with moderate salt restriction. Often these drugs are compounds that promote the elimination of salt and water from the body through the kidneys (diuretics), reducing the amount of sodium in the body by prompting its excretion rather than by drastically reducing its intake. Such treatment has markedly improved the life expectancy of persons, with hypertension, giving them, in fact, a normal life expectancy as long as their blood pressure is kept within the normal range.

SENILITY

Perhaps the most devastating and certainly the most feared consequence of aging is senility—the progressive degeneration of the nervous system that can impair the memory and often curtails the ability to perform even simple tasks. No treatment exists for senility and there is no known way to prevent it, despite the many remedies touted for this purpose. However, some recent research in nutrition and its effects on the nervous system—although not yet at a stage in which it might yield any treatment for senility in the near future—is interesting both because it may lead to new insights into the problem of senility and because it gives the lie to some popular claims.

In theory, one of the reasons for the changes that occur with senility is that aging results in a degeneration of many of the nerve-cell connections necessary for memory, coordinated thinking, and coordinated activity. Since nerve cells transmit messages to one another with chemicals that they produce and secrete, it has been reasoned that increasing the quantity of these chemical messengers would permit nerve cells to transmit messages to one another more readily, enabling the brain to compensate for the effects of aging on its cells. One of the most important chemicals in this regard is a substance called acetylcholine, which is made from another substance, known as choline, that is found in many foods. Furthermore, during the past few years, research at the Massachusetts Institute of Technology has shown that the amount of acetylcholine in the brain is directly related to the amount of choline consumed in the diet. Therefore, increasing the amount of choline in the diet will increase the amount of acetylcholine in the brain. As a result, lecithin (a compound made up largely of choline) has been tried experimentally in a number of nervous-system diseases including senility. But while such experiments have shown some promise in the treatment of certain conditions, they have not had any effect in patients with senility. No long-term treatment with choline has been tried in an attempt to prevent senility, since there is no experimental evidence that it works in this condition and no theoretical reason why it should work.

Yet despite these negative findings, expensive lecithin preparations are being sold over the counter with claims that they will prevent senility and lessen its consequences in those already suffering from it. This is more than simple misinformation; it is a cruel hoax played on aging persons who may understandably try any promised prevention or remedy for senility in themselves or their loved ones. Thus, while it may be important to be willing to try new things if the evidence warrants, it is equally important to be constantly vigilant for false claims made by modern health hucksters.

NUTRITIONAL REQUIREMENTS FOR OLDER WOMEN

With aging, just as with growth in childhood, the nutritional requirements for good health change in both men and women. While women's calcium requirements remain higher than men's, the need for such nutrients as iron, zinc and folic acid, which have been particularly important through middle age, becomes similar in both sexes. And women's other nutritional needs also approach those of men.

As logical as this may seem, it has only recently been recognized by the scientific community. The 1980 edition of the *Recommended Dietary Allowances* was the first to carry specific recommendations for older people, and many of these recommendations are still tentative and will probably have to be modified. But at least we have made a start. Yet the realization of the special nutritional needs of older persons has spurred great interest and activity among nutritional scientists, with the result that new information is becoming available almost daily in a number of scientific journals.

But this is a book on nutrition for women, and because of trends in longevity in the United States, as we have already seen, most older people in this country are women. Among people between 65 and 74 there are 1.4 women to each man; by age 80 that number reaches 1.8, and by 90 it reaches 2.5. This is one major reason why, when we discuss the nutritional requirements of older people, we are discussing a subject with special relevance to women.

Perhaps the best way to approach the change in nutritional requirements during aging is to examine what happens to certain body functions that are important to the maintenance of adequate nutrition. For one thing, aging, for most persons, means getting fatter. This is not because we gain weight, but rather because we lose muscle and other nonfat tissues. Thus, even older people who lose weight are relatively more obese than they were before. Second, the body's metabolism undergoes certain changes that result in a reduced need for calories. Finally, many older persons are less active than at earlier stages in their lives and therefore expend fewer calories. The net result of all of this is a decreased requirement for dietary calories. The exact amount of this decrease will vary from one person to another, but a good rule of thumb is that you will need about 10 percent fewer calories for your size and weight than when you were younger.

As far as the major nutrients are concerned, the best available evidence suggests that the body's protein requirements do not change with aging, but that the high quantities of protein in the typical American diet may cause problems for elderly persons. We have already seen one reason for this: excess protein promotes calcium loss from the bones. The second reason for a moderate protein intake is that the aging kidney cannot easily excrete the nitrogen-containing waste products that are produced by the digestion and metabolism of large amounts of protein. For these two reasons, it is recommended that elderly persons keep their dietary protein intake barely above the minimum requirement for protein, and that they use high-quality, easily digestible protein sources. Chicken, fish, dairy products and protein-containing vegetables are often best for this.

With regard to fat, the recommendation for elderly persons is not markedly different from that for younger people: the dietary fat intake should be reduced from the typical levels of nearly 50 percent of the calories in the American diet to about 30 percent of the total daily calorie intake. However, even though this recommendation is the same as for younger persons, the reasons for it are somewhat different: heart disease and cancer of the breast are of less concern to older women than to middle-aged and younger women; women who have entered their later years, particularly those in their seventies or above, have successfully passed the age of peak incidence of these diseases. They are in a sense survivors, and are much less likely to experience any further increase in the risk of developing these diseases. The major reason for the need of elderly persons to reduce their fat intake is to reduce their calories, of which fat is a major source.

How can this reduction in dietary fat be accomplished? Let us take an example. Suppose you currently have a daily dietary intake of 2,200 calories: 900 from fat, 450 from protein and 850 from carbohydrates. If you reduce your calorie intake by about 10 percent (to around 2,000) and reduce your protein intake to the minimum required (the amount that will provide about 15 percent of your calories), you will be getting 300 calories per day from protein sources. If you then increase the carbohydrate content of your diet to the level at about 55 percent of your calories—which is a desirable level—you will be getting 1,100 calories in the form of carbohydrates. This leaves 600 calories (a little more than 30 percent) to be derived from fat. Since for elderly persons the type of fat consumed is less important than for younger individuals, most of it can come from the fish, fowl and vegetable sources that provide the necessary protein in your diet. Much of this fat is unsaturated fat. If your diet contains more meat and dairy foods, you will be consuming more saturated fat. In either case, don't worry. You have lived past the age of major risk, and whatever fat you eat is perfectly acceptable as long as your total fat intake is around 30 percent of your total caloric intake.

As was mentioned above, about 55 percent of your calories should come from carbohydrates, and mainly from complex carbohydrates—the best sources of which are grains, cereals, vegetables and certain fruits. There are three reasons for this relatively high carbohydrate recommendation. First, the complex carbohydrates are nutrient dense; they are the major source of many of the micronutrients whose requirements may increase in older people. Second, with aging, the gastrointestinal tract can handle complex carbohydrates better than either protein or fat. In fact, dietary fiber, which is a major component of complex carbohydrate foods, is specifically beneficial to the gastrointestinal tract in elderly persons in that it eases elimination and can prevent constipation and some of its more serious consequences. Finally, part of the aging process is that the ability to metabolize simple sugars—such as refined sugar—is impaired. The digestion of complex carbohydrates, in contrast to simple sugars, will release sugar into the blood far more slowly, and will therefore cause much less marked changes in the blood sugar level.

One specific change that occurs in the gastrointestinal tract with aging is a loss of mobility. The muscles in the tract cannot contract as efficiently as they formerly could, and as a result food is not moved along the tract as rapidly. When this occurs, water is absorbed and the stool becomes harder. This leads to constipation, a frequent discomfort among older persons. Furthermore, the bowel must work harder, generating increased pressure, to move the hardened, dehydrated waste contents of digestion through it, with the result that weak areas of the bowel may be forced outward, in the form of small "pockets" or swellings. These outpouchings are called diverticuli, and their occurrence in large numbers leads to a condition called diverticulosis which is virtually unknown in younger persons. The diverticuli may then collect debris from the passing intestinal contents, and often become infected. The condition that results when this happens is called diverticulitis, which may be accompanied by very severe symptoms of

acute abdominal pain, nausea and vomiting and often requires immediate medical attention and sometimes surgery. When it is considered that approximately 20 percent
of persons over the age of seventy have diverticulosis—a
population conservatively including two million women—
we can see that chronic constipation is a serious problem
in older women. By far the best approach to preventing
this problem and its effects is a high dietary fiber content.

Wheat and other grain brans are major types of dietary
fiber; the pectin in apples and other fruits is another, while
many vegetables provide yet other types of fiber. The
human intestine cannot digest this fiber, and it therefore
passes through the intestine in undigested form. As it
passes through the gastrointestinal tract, the fiber traps
water, rendering the contents of the tract softer and decreasing the pressure and increasing the rate at which these
contents are moved along and out of the tract. Constipation
is relieved and the tendency to develop diverticuli is reduced.

Furthermore, while the evidence for this is less compelling, there are indications that fiber may be important in
reducing the incidence of several other serious problems
that are common among older persons. Chief among these
is cancer of the colon, which according to current theory
is caused by a combination of two factors: a high dietary fat
content and a low dietary fiber content occurring for a long
time. It is known that diets with a high fat content promote
the formation of breakdown products within the intestine
and that many of these products are capable of inducing
cancer. Moreover, the longer these products remain in contact with the cells that line the intestinal tract, the greater
is the chance for these cells to become cancerous. Thus,
since in older persons the contents of the intestine move
more slowly, the longer is the period over which such
contact occurs, and the greater is the risk of a cancer origi-

nating. This is where fiber plays its part. Diets with a high fiber content increase the rate of movement of fats and other digestive breakdown products through the intestine and hence decrease the risk of cancer. The evidence for this effect, both from animal experiments and observations of human populations, is compelling. It is much more difficult to induce colon cancer in animals fed a low-fat, high-fiber diet than in animals whose diets are high in fat and low in fiber. Additionally, in many rural parts of Africa, where the diet is very high in fiber and very low in fat, cancer of the colon is virtually unknown, while the movement of people from these regions to urban centers and a more Western, higher fat, lower fiber diet results in a growing incidence of colon cancer. Thus, in combining the recommendation for a reduction in dietary fat with that for an increase in dietary fiber both in older persons and in those of any other age group, not only are separate benefits derived, but the combination may offer specific protection against colon cancer.

OTHER CHANGES IN THE GASTROINTESTINAL TRACT

Besides a reduced motility, a number of other gastrointestinal-tract changes that accompany aging influence the nutritional requirements of older persons. Since a very large number of such persons either have false teeth or are missing a significant number of teeth, they may either be unable to eat hard foods, or such foods may create problems that lead to their avoidance. Twenty percent of the baby foods sold in this country are consumed by the elderly. Clearly, this does not constitute a solution to the problem; were the food industry to create wholesome food products of the proper consistency and portion size for older buyers, it would be making a real contribution to the nutritional needs of Americans. Lacking this, the blender can be a great help for those who cannot chew hard foods.

With aging, the stomach undergoes two changes that affect the nutrient requirements of the body: it secretes less acid than in younger persons and it makes less of a particular protein called intrinsic factor. The acid that the stomach secretes is necessary for initiating the digestion of a number of foods, and the digestion of these foods may therefore be a problem for some older persons. Meats, and particularly red meats, fall into this category, as do certain vegetables. Additionally, the acid made by the stomach is necessary for converting dietary iron into a form that the body can absorb. Consequently, elderly persons must be attentive to the iron content in their diets, and this is true for women even after they have passed their menopause and no longer lose large quantities of iron every month. However, this does not present the problem that it does at the earlier stages in a woman's life, since her overall iron requirements will have decreased, and if she is not depleted and continues to eat foods with a high iron content, she should have no trouble.

Intrinsic factor is a protein made in the stomach that couples with vitamin B_{12} to permit the absorption of the vitamin into the body. Because its production decreases with age, older persons must give special attention to meeting their vitamin B_{12} requirements, since a shortage of the vitamin, when combined with its decreased absorption, can lead to deficiency. If meat and dairy products are already a significant part of your diet you need not worry. You are likely to be getting plenty of vitamin B_{12}. But if, on the other hand, your diet consists almost entirely of fruits, vegetables and grains you will need a supply of vitamin B_{12}. This can come from small amounts of meat, fish, fowl or dairy products, from fortified foods or from oral supplements of the vitamin. Beware of the use of injections of vitamin B_{12}; they have their use (for example, following stomach surgery) but are generally not needed by older persons.

The precise requirements for the other vitamins and minerals in older persons have not been established. We do not know whether the changes in metabolism that accompany aging affect the requirements for most of these nutrients, and the requirements for most vitamins and minerals are therefore currently considered to be the same for older persons as for young adults. Despite this, some new evidence suggests that such an assumption may not be valid. For example, at least one trace element, chromium, may be needed in greater amounts in older persons. The only known function of chromium in the body is as part of a yet undefined factor that aids the body in metabolizing glucose, the sugar that is its main fuel. It has been found that rats made deficient in chromium develop an impaired ability to metabolize glucose and show signs and symptoms identical to those of mild diabetes. It is also known that older persons have lower levels of chromium in their serum and in other tissues, and that many older persons have an impaired glucose metabolism similar to that seen in chromium-deficient rats. With regard to this, various studies have shown that chromium supplements to the diet, either in the form of tablets or in brewer's yeast, which is rich in chromium, frequently improves glucose metabolism in such cases.

Thus, while the information about chromium in the human diet is still incomplete, the use of brewer's yeast in moderate amounts presents no problem, and may enhance the body's capacity to metabolize glucose. As far as direct chromium supplementation is concerned, very small amounts are more than adequate, and since we do not yet know whether there are any dangers in the prolonged use of chromium supplements, they should be used only under a doctor's advice and supervision.

DRUG NUTRIENT INTERACTIONS

One of the most important aspects of aging, from the nutritional standpoint, is the increased consumption of drugs that is common among older persons. In part, this is due to the increased frequency of illness seen in the elderly population, and in part to the feelings of weakness, tiredness and other nonspecific symptoms that typically accompany aging. Unfortunately, despite their beneficial effects in many cases, a good many of the drugs taken by older persons can interfere with the absorption or metabolism of various nutrients and thereby change the requirements for these nutrients. The first rule to follow, therefore, is to take only those drugs that are necessary for your health. Second, if you must take a drug, find out if it can in any way affect your nutritional requirements and if so, how. Third, always check with your doctor if you plan to take a drug, even a seemingly innocuous drug, for any period of time. In the following sections I will discuss only certain of the drugs used by older persons, but the above rules apply to all drugs.

We have already seen that in the American population blood pressure increases with age, and that many older people therefore suffer from hypertension. The most common way of treating this is with the combination of a sodium-restricted diet and drugs. The type of drug most often used is known as a diuretic, which has the effect of making the kidney excrete increased quantities of both water and sodium from the body, thereby reducing the blood pressure. The water that is lost with the use of a diuretic should be replaced by consuming somewhat more fluid—a situation which ordinarily presents no problem since the thirst mechanism automatically controls the body's fluid needs and intake. However, besides promoting a loss of sodium and water, many diuretics also cause the body to lose another mineral, potassium, which is a very important nutrient since it constitutes the major mineral in every cell in the body. Therefore, if you are using a diuretic to control your blood pressure, you should pay special attention to getting foods rich in potassium. Table 3 gives a list of such foods.

TABLE 3 FOODS WITH A HIGH POTASSIUM CONTENT

DAIRY PRODUCTS
    Milk (regular, skim and low sodium)
    Eggs
SWEETS
    Brown, packed sugar
JUICES
    Apricot, grapefruit, orange, prune, tomato
VEGETABLES
    Asparagus, broccoli, carrots, potato, tomato
FRUITS
    Bananas, apricots, oranges, peaches, pears

Occasionally, the use of a diuretic may produce a potassium loss great enough to warrant direct potassium supplementation. Your doctor will tell you if this is necessary.

Aspirin is a drug that many people consider to be totally harmless, and which is used in huge amounts by older people, particularly for arthritis. Yet it can and does irritate the gastrointestinal tract, especially in older persons, and can cause microscopic, unnoticeable bleeding. Over a long period this can result in iron deficiency, which as we have seen is particularly prevalent among older women. Thus, if you must take aspirin—and some people must—you should pay special attention to getting a sufficient amount of iron in your diet.

Antacids are another group of drugs widely used by older persons. Part of the reason for this is the widespread occurrence of "heartburn"—which many older persons perceive as being caused by excess gastric acid—in this age group. This perception is reenforced by advertisements showing how much acid one or another antacid can neutralize. With regard to this, it is worth recalling that one of the major changes in the stomach that occurs with aging is a loss of the ability to make acid, with the result that older people suffer from a deficiency of stomach acid, not an excess. Therefore, particularly for older people, there is little reason to use antacids. If you do use them, and especially if you use them regularly, because they contain certain minerals and phosphorus, you run the risk of causing an increased loss of calcium from your bones and upsetting the balance of several other important nutrients. As far as heartburn is concerned, it is caused by a regurgitation of partially digested food from the stomach into the lower esophagus, as a result of the weakening with age of the valve between the two. Smaller, more frequent meals, eaten more slowly, will usually solve the problem.

Other drugs have their own undesirable effects. Thus, if you must take a drug, ask your physician if there is any reason to pay particular attention to one or more aspects of your nutrition.

Good nutrition for an older woman does not entail radical changes in her eating pattern, particularly if this pattern has generally been good since her middle years. Furthermore, even if such a radical change were called for, it would not be easily implemented, since older people tend to like the same foods they did when younger. What may be very important to an older person, however, are changes in nutritional emphasis. Thus, an older woman should give careful attention to meeting her dietary calcium, phosphorus and protein needs, and should also see that she gets enough complex carbohydrate, with its rich supply of micronutrients and fiber. Salt should be avoided, even by persons for whom a slow loss of taste with aging makes certain foods taste bland. There are many other ways to season foods, and many alternative foods. Additionally, since older people consume more drugs than younger ones, they must protect themselves against potentially damaging interactions of drugs and nutrients. Finally, because women constitute a greater part of the elderly population than men, all of these considerations involve women to a greater extent than men. Yet there is no doubt that the moderate dietary alterations discussed here are a small price to pay for the extra years a woman can expect to add to her life.

CHAPTER 9

Diseases Common to Women

So far, we have dealt with the role of nutrition in maintaining a woman's health. But no matter how good our nutrition, we all get sick sometime in life. Yet many illnesses, and even those not caused by poor dietary patterns, can be at least partially treated through nutrition. In this chapter we will discuss some of the illnesses that most commonly affect women and in whose treatment nutrition plays an important role. Since we have already covered such illnesses as hypertension, diverticulitis and osteoporosis, whose incidence can be reduced by proper nutritional patterns, we will not further discuss them here. Nor, because we have already covered it in detail in various contexts and in relation to the different stages in a woman's life cycle, will we discuss obesity.

Thus, the diseases that are discussed in the following sections are not meant to constitute a complete list of the diseases that may affect women; rather, they all have two things in common: they are more frequent or more serious in women than in men, and they are all at least partially amenable to proper nutrition. For easy reference I will discuss these diseases in their alphabetical order, and hence their location among the following sections in no way indicates either their frequency or their importance.

ALCOHOLISM

Although alcoholism is more common among men than among women, it is a greater health risk for women. We have already discussed its effects on the absorption of various nutrients that are in short supply in many women's diets, and we have seen that alcohol consumed during pregnancy may be toxic to the developing fetus. But alcohol is also more toxic to women themselves than to men: it has been estimated that a 20 percent smaller quantity of alcohol than that required for men will produce cirrhosis—a serious and often fatal liver disease—in women. The metabolic factor that makes women more susceptible to such toxic effects of alcohol has not yet been identified. Nevertheless, the incidence of alcoholism among women is increasing. Therefore, if you have a drinking problem, the first rule is to get help. At the same time—to ensure that while you are under treatment for the primary condition you do not develop secondary nutritional deficiencies—pay close attention to good nutrition. Eat a varied diet, with an emphasis on foods high in folic acid, vitamin B_6, thiamine (vitamin B_1) and zinc—especially green leafy vegetables, whole grains, meat and fish—and supplement it daily with multivitamins and minerals.

ANEMIA

The term "anemia" simply means that the blood lacks enough hemoglobin to carry the necessary amount of oxygen from the lungs to the rest of the body, and to carry carbon dioxide back from the cells to be exhaled by the lungs. And because iron is the vital structural component of hemoglobin, a lack of iron will result in a shortage of this essential substance, even though hemoglobin contains protein as well as iron. In fact, the body's manufacture of hemoglobin can be compared to the making of concrete: no matter how much sand you have, you can't make any more concrete if you run out of cement. But while iron deficiency anemia is the most common nutritionally caused disease among American women, anemia may be caused by lack of other nutrients or by problems that have nothing to do with nutrition.

All of the body's functional hemoglobin is packaged in the small, round red cells of the blood, which—in contrast to most of the body's cells—contain no nucleus. The red cells are efficient in their task of carrying oxygen and carbon dioxide, but in order to achieve that efficiency they have sacrificed the longevity characteristic of most other cells, and have an average lifespan of only 120 days. Thus, about 1 percent of your red cells die each day, and must be replaced. They are replaced by cells formed in the bone marrow, which serves as a factory for the production of new red cells. There, a type of nucleated cell that is a "precursor" of the red cell undergoes continuous division, giving rise to new red cells which then mature into "adult" red cells, losing their nuclei in the process. The rate at which the precursor cells divide is partly controlled by the rate at which red cells die and are lost from the blood, and any condition that causes red cells to die more rapidly than normal will therefore result in a more rapid rate of division of the precursor cells within the bone marrow.

As can be seen from this discussion, bleeding is one condition that causes red cells to be lost at a more rapid rate than normal, and because women bleed with every menstrual period, their bone marrow is more active during the years from puberty to menopause than is the bone marrow of men. Moreover, the heavier a woman's menstrual periods, the more active her bone marrow will be in replacing the red cells she loses. However, in order for the precursor cells in the marrow to maintain an adequate rate of division into new red cells, the raw materials necessary for cell division must be available in greater amounts. As we have already seen, the most important of these raw materials are zinc, folic acid and vitamin B_{12}; a shortage of any of these three nutrients will result in a slowing of the rate of cell division and hence an inability to replace all of the lost red cells. Furthermore, if this situation continues for any length of time (weeks to months), the number of red cells in the blood will gradually diminish. Under such circumstances—even if enough iron is available to manufacture hemoglobin—there will not be enough red cells to carry this hemoglobin, and the iron that would be used in the hemoglobin will instead remain in the body's storage depots. The overall result will be an inadequate amount of hemoglobin in the blood, or anemia.

Thus, anemia may be caused by anything that increases red cell destruction or decreases red cell production—a situation that includes literally dozens of medical conditions.

Whatever its cause, anemia will show itself as a group of symptoms related to the decreased hemoglobin content of the blood. First—since hemoglobin has a reddish color when it is carrying oxygen, and it is this color that imparts the pinkish tinge to the skin—a reduced amount of hemoglobin will result in a pale appearance that is most obvious in areas where the blood comes nearest to the skin surface, such as the finger- and toenail beds, the inside lining of the mouth, the lips and the thin skin around the eyes. To a trained eye this "paleness" will be visible in people of all races and all complexions.

The other symptoms of anemia result directly from the

inability of the limited amount of hemoglobin to do its job properly. At first these symptoms—including tiredness, sluggishness and irritability—may be barely perceptible. As the anemia worsens, however, genuine fatigue may set in, with a decreasing ability to concentrate that may affect a child's school performance or an adult's performance on the job. Finally, anemia may produce exhaustion with the least amount of exertion, and a rapid shortness of breath.

In addition to the general symptoms of anemia discussed above, anemia caused by a lack of iron, zinc, folic acid or vitamin B_{12} will be accompanied by other signs and symptoms. For example, zinc deficiency, besides causing anemia, can result in poor growth and immature sexual development as well as abnormalities in taste. Folic acid deficiency may result in abnormal vaginal and cervical skin, and prolonged vitamin B_{12} deficiency may lead to severe and permanent damage to the nervous system.

Practically speaking, what this means is that a lasting feeling of tiredness or irritability could come from anemia. A rapid test by your physician, on a drop of blood from your finger, will reveal whether in fact you are anemic, and if so, will frequently reveal the cause of the anemia as well. And most often, if the cause is nutritional, so is the cure. Thus, iron-deficiency anemia requires iron, and only iron will cure it. Similarly, many women are deficient in iron and folic acid, and a successful cure of the anemia requires both of these nutrients. On the other hand, many women who feel tired or irritable are not deficient in iron or folic acid, and hence neither of these two nutrients will affect these symptoms. In fact, since anemia may sometimes be a symptom of a more serious, non-nutritional illness, it is important that you be carefully examined by a physician for any of the symptoms named above.

For all of the foregoing reasons—and despite the television and radio commercials constantly encouraging us to take this tonic or that pill for this or that run-down feeling or "tired blood"—consult your physician and find out why you are truly tired and run down. If your symptoms are due to a nutritional deficiency, it can easily be corrected either dietarily or by direct supplementation. If your fatigue does not come from this, you will have saved valuable time and money that would have been wasted in trying to cure a condition that doesn't exist.

ANOREXIA

In some girls, the adolescent fixation on weight and body image can take an extreme form, with potentially serious consequences. The self-image of being "fat" can prompt a weight reduction so severe that it impairs health and may lead to starvation and, ultimately, death. The condition characterized by such near starvation, profound weight loss, emaciation and serious nutritional deficiencies is confined almost exclusively to adolescent girls and is called anorexia nervosa. It is brought about by voluntary food restriction, often aggravated by self-induced vomiting and sometimes by the ingestion of diuretic pills to promote water loss from the body. There is an obsessive concern with weight. The youngster is constantly on and off the scale and no matter how thin she is never feels that she is thin enough. As the condition progresses, weight loss becomes so severe that the youngster appears emaciated, with almost no visible fat tissue, her growth ceases and certain body functions are affected; she will constantly feel cold and her body temperature may drop; her blood pressure and heart rate will fall below normal, sometimes dangerously so. Her blood sugar concentration may also decrease and the concentration of certain minerals in her blood may be very low.

Obviously any youngster with this problem in its full-blown form has serious psychological problems that must be dealt with simultaneously with the nutritional deficiencies caused by the condition. However, the nutritional deficiencies may take precedence, since they are the ones most acutely threatening to life.

The youngster suffering from anorexia should therefore be brought under experienced medical care, which usually means a team consisting of a pediatrician or internist and a psychiatrist experienced in dealing with the condition.

The treatment is often a complicated matter, entailing correcting the nutritional deficiencies, usually over some time, since the youngster will ordinarily not cooperate initially. At the same time the psychiatric treatment seeks to eradicate the cause of the illness. Anorexia is not a condition which the family should attempt to deal with itself; the stakes are too high.

Most health professionals who care for young women with anorexia believe that its frequency among adolescent girls is increasing rapidly, whereas twenty or thirty years ago it was rarely seen. Perhaps what is most alarming is that milder forms of anorexia are becoming more frequent among teen-age girls. The usual case history is that of an adolescent girl who has actually been overweight or who has perceived herself as being such and who begins to diet, often with parental encouragement. The latest fad diet is usually tried and works, with the girl losing weight but— as is often the case—with the weight rapidly returning when the diet ends. She then tries the next diet, which has reached the top of the best-seller list just in time. Again she loses weight only to regain it rapidly. Frustration sets in and her fixation on controlling her weight continues. Support from the family begins to erode as they show their disappointment. Slowly, the youngster's sense of reality becomes distorted and she begins to think of herself only as a fat person, and disliking herself intensely for it. Fortu-

nately, most girls with this history get through adolescence
and enter adulthood. Many, however, leave adolescence as
extremely thin individuals, and may continue their obses-
sion for thinness for many years and even for the rest of
their lives.

Certain signs should alert the family that a youngster's
restrictive eating pattern is becoming potentially dangerous. One cause for concern is a child who is obviously
underweight yet clearly sees herself as fat. Medical help
should be sought immediately for a youngster who vomits
frequently or has taken to using pills to "get rid of excess
water." The same is true if the girl's growth stops, if she
complains of feeling cold, gets dizzy or faints frequently or
cannot maintain her former activity level. If in doubt consult your physician.

On the other hand, the family, friends and health professionals caring for a child who is obviously overconcerned
with weight control but who does not manifest the symptoms of anorexia can often provide the support necessary
to get her through a very difficult period in her life. In
order to do this, however, they must realize that a problem
exists and that putting too much pressure on the youngster,
particularly if she fails, may aggravate the problem. Sometimes the parents are more fixed on the child's being thin
than is the child herself, especially if they are under social,
media, and "success oriented" pressures. In such cases a
"fat" child may subconsciously embarrass them, and they
may overreact and transmit their own—often unrealistic—
fears to the child. Remember, realistic goals should be set
and once reached should be maintained. A child who
reaches a reasonable weight-loss goal should be praised and
encouraged to maintain her newly attained appearance.
Finally, the parents and the child must realize that time—
and sometimes a long time—is necessary for this.

ARTHRITIS

Arthritis is an inflammation of one or more of the body's joints. The two most common forms of the condition are rheumatoid arthritis and osteoarthritis. Both are more common in women than in men, and both have nutritional implications.

Rheumatoid arthritis affects one person in a hundred and is about three times more common in women than in men. It usually begins between the ages of thirty-five and forty-five. Often the onset is sudden, with simultaneous swelling and pain in several joints. The most commonly affected joints are the small joints of the hands and feet, the wrists, the elbows and the ankles. Early morning stiffness and pain are frequent symptoms of rheumatoid arthritis. The disease may result in severe disability and if untreated can lead to permanent joint deformities.

Although there is no specific nutritional treatment for rheumatoid arthritis, nutrition does play an important role in the overall management of the disease. For example, physicians who treat rheumatoid arthritis usually prescribe large doses of aspirin four times a day, which should be consumed with or just after food even if the aspirin is taken in a buffered form. If you are on such a regimen you should therefore divide your eating into three meals and a bedtime snack. This will help to keep the acidity of the stomach at a minimum, and hence keep the aspirin (which is an acid) from irritating the stomach. Foods high in protein, such as dairy products, meat and fish, are very helpful in this respect. Even with these precautions, however, aspirin may cause chronic bleeding from the gastrointestinal tract. Since such bleeding can result in iron deficiency, it is important to eat a diet rich in iron and to have your blood checked frequently if you are being treated with aspirin for rheumatoid arthritis.

Other, more potent drugs are sometimes used to treat rheumatoid arthritis when aspirin alone cannot control the pain and inflammation. One of these drugs, d-penicillamine, is a very potent and potentially dangerous agent that should be taken only under the careful supervision of a physician. Among the side effects of d-penicillamine is that it interferes with the absorption of vitamin B_6. Because this can lead to depression and other nervous symptoms, any person taking d-penicillamine should also take a vitamin B_6 supplement.

For some reason, rheumatoid arthritis is a favorite disease among nutritional hucksters. Beware of claims that this amino acid or that vitamin or mineral will offer instant relief from the symptoms of this condition. None of these claims has any basis in fact.

Unlike rheumatoid arthritis, osteoarthritis usually affects the body's weight-bearing joints. The symptoms are pain, especially when an affected joint is made to bear weight or put under some type of stress. The incidence of osteoarthritis increases with age, and after the age of forty-five it is much more common among women than among men. Osteoarthritis also occurs more frequently in obese people, and the obesity aggravates the disease. If you have osteoarthritis and are overweight, it is therefore important that you reduce. Even if you are only a bit overweight the loss of a few pounds will help. Additionally, persons with osteoarthritis must frequently cut down on certain athletic activities since these may make the condition worse. However, this does not mean that you should be sedentary, since this will only aggravate your weight problem and increase the rate of calcium loss from your body, which can lead to osteoporosis. A good insurance against calcium depletion is a diet of calcium-rich foods or the use of a calcium supplement. This will not help in treating the osteoarthritis itself, but may slow the process of chronic calcium loss.

BED REST

One of the most common aspects of the treatment of many diseases is bed rest. In the case of a chronic disease and certain surgically treated conditions, the period of bed rest may be prolonged. Although women as a group do not require more prolonged periods of time in bed for illness than men, prolonged bed rest can result in the loss of calcium from the bones, which is a more serious condition for women than for men. Therefore, if you must spend considerable time in bed recovering from an illness, be sure to do the maximum amount of activity permitted out of bed. Even while you are in bed it is important to move around as much as possible and exercise your muscles, as long as this is allowed. Finally, if you must be immobilized for more than a few days, it is important to have a diet high in calcium and to consume a calcium supplement.

BULIMIA

Bulimia, a condition usually affecting young women, is characterized by alternating food binges and purges. It is thought by some to be related to anorexia nervosa because both conditions are marked by an unreasonable fear of becoming fat and a distorted body image.

However, while persons with anorexia generally avoid food, those with bulimia first gorge themselves and then purge the food they have eaten through vomiting or the use of laxatives. Another important difference is that persons close to a young woman with anorexia are usually aware of the problem since the victim becomes obviously thin and emaciated, whereas bulimia is generally characterized by elaborate secrecy, frequently to the point at which even the closest relatives of the affected person are not aware of it. Nor, frequently, are there any outward clues to the disorder, since the alternate gorging and purging frequently leaves the bulimic individual close to her proper weight.

The most dangerous medical complications of bulimia are heart or kidney failure caused by fluid and mineral losses from the self-induced vomiting or diarrhea. Additionally, general dehydration, liver damage, stomach rupture, swollen salivary glands, chronic sore throat, inflammation of the esophagus and a number of other medical conditions may occur. Finally, bulimia can lead to severe deficiencies of iron, folic acid, zinc and other nutrients. Calcium deficiency may also result and may manifest itself in the form of devastating tooth decay, caused by a combination of stomach acid eroding the teeth and shortages of calcium and vitamin D preventing their reconstruction.

If you know someone with bulimia, urge or take her to get help. The earlier the treatment is started the better the outcome. A team approach involving a physician, nutritionist, psychotherapist and social worker is often successful. Sometimes behavior modification therapy is used. As soon as control of the symptoms has begun, nutritional rehabilitation, including the use of vitamin and mineral supplements, should be undertaken. A good place to seek treatment is at a center that cares for people with anorexia nervosa. Most centers that deal with adolescents have had experience with this disease. Unfortunately, bulimia, like anorexia, is becoming much more common in today's weight-conscious environment.

DEPRESSION

Feelings of dejection and despair from such adverse experiences as bereavement, the breaking up of a relationship or a career setback can sometimes reach a state that can be out of proportion to the precipitating stress. A severe depression may seriously compromise a person's ability to function.

Although depression affects both men and women, it is more common among women, particularly during certain periods of their lives. After delivery, for example, some women experience a depression that usually lasts for only a short time. In a few, however, this postpartum depression may persist for months or even longer. Menopause is another period during which depression is common.

A nutritional source of nervous symptoms, including depression, is a deficiency of certain vitamins, and particularly vitamin B_6. This may be why high doses of certain B vitamins have been suggested in the treatment of depression. Generally, however, this form of treatment does not work. Nevertheless, since many women, and particularly those using contraceptive pills, may be deficient in vitamin B_6, and since such a deficiency can aggravate the symptoms of depression, there is no harm in the use of a B-complex vitamin supplement for women who are under such circumstances and who are also depressed.

GALL-BLADDER DISEASE

Gall-bladder disease is much more common among women—and particularly those under fifty—than among men. It is also much more frequent in obese women than in those of normal weight. It usually begins with the formation of small stones produced by the collection and hardening of cholesterol from the bile. These stones may obstruct the flow of bile and create an inflammation of the gall bladder. The symptoms of this can include acute pain, usually in the right side of the abdomen, which may be accompanied by nausea and vomiting. Chronic dull pain, particularly after a fatty meal, is another common symptom.

There is some evidence that low fiber diets are related to gall-bladder disease. This, and the association of the disease with obesity, means that there is a strong nutritional component in the cause of gall-bladder disease. Because of this, weight reduction and a high-fiber diet play an important role in reducing the risk of the disease.

From the standpoint of treating gall-bladder disease, a low-fat diet is often advocated, since fat stimulates the secretion of bile—which is necessary for the digestion of fat —and the contraction of the gall bladder that is necessary for this secretion. Because other aspects of treatment of the disease involve drugs and sometimes surgery, anyone with gall-bladder disease should be under the care of a physician.

GESTATIONAL DIABETES

Diabetes is a serious disease in which the pancreas, an organ located behind the liver, cannot produce enough of the hormone insulin to regulate the metabolism of glucose (the main sugar used by the body). As a result of the pancreas's inability to produce a normal quantity of insulin, the hallmark of diabetes is a high level of glucose in the blood. The disease occurs with equal frequency in men and women, and its effects and complications make it equally severe in both sexes. Occasionally diabetes makes its first appearance during pregnancy. This form of diabetes is called gestational diabetes. The control of diabetes usually involves supplying insulin to the body in the form of one or more daily injections of this hormone and a proper diet.

Any woman who is diabetic, whether she has had the disease since before pregnancy or whether it began during that time, has a greater than normal risk both in terms of her own health and in terms of the development of her fetus. Infants of diabetic mothers have a higher mortality, are more often born with congenital malformations and growth abnormalities, and are more likely to have problems in the immediate period after birth than are those born to women unaffected by the disease.

It is the high blood-sugar level that adversely affects the fetus in women who have diabetes. Exactly how this happens is not fully understood, but it is well known that the better the control of the level of the mother's blood sugar the better the outcome for the fetus. Today most women with well-controlled diabetes can expect to have a normal infant.

If you have diabetes and are pregnant your physician will aim at balancing your diet and your insulin treatments to achieve blood sugar levels that are within the normal range throughout the day. Usually, this can at least be closely approximated with careful medical supervision.

The diet of a woman who is pregnant and has diabetes is one that should contain sufficient calories for her fetus to grow normally, should consist of properly spaced meals to help keep her blood sugar levels from getting too high or too low, should be low in fat and simple sugar and should be high in complex carbohydrates. The same rules about getting enough vitamins and minerals hold for the pregnant woman with diabetes as for those without this illness. The rules for the calorie content of the diet are no different than those for pregnant women who do not have diabetes. However, since insulin is not being provided in sufficient amounts by the pancreas, which normally secretes insulin in response to an increased blood sugar level, the food intake should be spaced in such a way as to coincide with the peak activity of the insulin treatments. Usually, three regular meals per day accompanied by a midmorning, late afternoon and before-bedtime snack will accomplish this. An important aspect of the diet is that it should have a high content of complex carbohydrates, such as bread, pasta or rice, since these sources release sugar slowly (to prevent wide swings in blood sugar levels) and because such foods are low in fat, which can be harmful if taken in excess. Simple sugars, particularly refined sugar, should be limited since they can rapidly increase the blood sugar concentration.

HIATUS HERNIA

A hiatus hernia occurs when part of the stomach protrudes through a weakness in the wall of the diaphragm. It is the most common type of structural abnormality of the upper gastrointestinal tract, and its frequency increases markedly with age. Thus, only 9 percent of persons under the age of forty have had this condition, whereas 69 percent of those over seventy are affected by it. And since the elderly population has many more women than men, hiatus hernia is more common among women than among men.

A hiatus hernia will often cause no discomfort. Sometimes, however, symptoms of heartburn may occur. This usually happens when some of the acid contents of the stomach are forced back up into the esophagus and irritate its lining. Occasionally pain, often described as a pressure, lump or fullness occurs. Such discomfort is often initiated or aggravated by a particularly large meal, emotional upset or physical exertion after eating.

Dietary management is an important component in the overall treatment of symptomatic hiatus hernia. Weight reduction is essential for overweight persons affected by the condition. This should be accomplished gradually. A low-fat diet is essential since fat tends to loosen the valve at the lower end of the esophagus, allowing the stomach contents to reflux into the esophagus. Meals should be small and frequent, and eating before retiring to bed should be avoided. It is a good idea for women with hiatus hernia to rest after meals.

The medical treatment of hiatus hernia often involves the use of antacids and other medications. These should be taken only under the specific direction of a physician. Their prolonged and unsupervised use may actually make the symptoms of the condition worse and can cause undesirable side effects. Women who experience night pain from the hernia often find it helpful to elevate the head of the bed. Such simple measures, with proper treatment will most often relieve the symptoms of hiatus hernia within a short time.

HYPOGLYCEMIA

Hypoglycemia is a condition from which many women think they suffer when in fact they do not; true hypoglycemia is very rare and must be diagnosed by a physician after appropriate tests. The diagnosis can be made only if a low blood sugar level (less than 40 mg of glucose per 100 ml of blood) occurs three to four hours after glucose is consumed and symptoms occur at the same time. Either criterion alone is not enough. What leads many women to believe they have the true condition are feelings of faintness, dizziness, palpitations, sweating and generalized weakness which usually occur three to four hours after a meal and in true hypoglycemia are brought on by the low blood sugar level at that time. In fact, however, these symptoms are not specific for hypoglycemia and can result from many other causes. Moreover, such symptoms of true hypoglycemia may not occur even when the levels of glucose in the blood are very low.

If you truly have hypoglycemia you will need to space your food intake carefully. A snack consisting of a complex carbohydrate food should be taken at midmorning, midafternoon and before going to bed. This will release sugar into your blood slowly and thereby prevent your blood sugar from falling too low. However, since hypoglycemia is often a symptom of more serious illness, such as early diabetes, you should not undertake such an eating plan on your own. Your doctor will want to eliminate all of the possible causes of your symptoms before recommending dietary treatment.

INJURY

Two types of injury—bleeding and broken bones—have special significance for women. Any significant blood loss from the body will result in an iron loss. The iron lost in internal bleeding, such as from a hemorrhage into a muscle, is reabsorbed by the body and can be reused by it, even though the blood loss itself can cause medical problems. The loss of one ounce of blood from the body means the loss of 15 milligrams of iron from the system (about one day's iron requirement), and a severe nosebleed can result in the loss of five to ten ounces of blood. Cuts are usually not this severe but they, too, can cause significant blood loss.

The iron that is lost in such injuries should be replaced rapidly with a diet rich in iron, including iron-fortified foods. If a large amount of blood has been lost, an iron supplement of twenty to thirty milligrams daily should be taken. It is a good idea also to seek foods that are high in folic acid, since the requirement for this vitamin will increase as the bone marrow becomes more active in making new red blood cells.

Broken bones are becoming much more frequent as both men and women engage more actively in a growing number of sports. Any fracture will increase the body's demand for calcium for rebuilding of the bone at the fracture site.

If this calcium is not provided in the diet it will be provided at the expense of the body's other bones. Additionally, the major treatment for a fractured bone is immobilization of the affected limb. Since this will lead to a loss of calcium in the unaffected bones in that limb, it is a second reason for a diet high in calcium and the use of a calcium supplement (500 milligrams per day). Furthermore, because any injury that results in a fracture will cause damage to the soft tissues, including some bleeding, both iron and folic acid replacement will be necessary, although the iron need will not be as critical as with external blood loss. Requirements for vitamin C will also increase since this nutrient is important in the healing process. Therefore citrus fruits and other good sources of vitamin C should be consumed. Remember, no injury is trivial.

THE IRRITABLE BOWEL SYNDROME (SPASTIC COLON)

Irritable bowel syndrome is another condition that occurs more commonly in women than in men, often in relation to periods of stress. There is no known organic cause of the condition. In some cases it is accompanied by depression. If the condition is severe it can be quite debilitating and psychotherapy may be necessary. The symptoms may vary but can usually be divided into two groups, the first of which, known as *spastic colon type* symptoms, usually includes severe pain over the lower abdomen with alternating periods of diarrhea and constipation. In the second group of symptoms the problem is primarily a painless diarrhea which is often urgent and which may occur on awaking in the morning and during or right after a meal.

There is no specific treatment for irritable bowel syndrome, but certain drugs may be useful in controlling the symptoms. Moreover, since any prolonged diarrhea will cause nutrient losses, and particularly the loss of those nutrients that are absorbed in the lower portion of the gastrointestinal tract, proper nutrition is extremely important in preventing certain nutrient deficiencies that can complicate the syndrome. For women with the syndrome, folic acid is important in this regard, as are sodium and potassium, which can also be lost. Finally, abdominal pain and diarrhea will cause a loss of appetite, which will contribute to deficiencies of various nutrients. Therefore, women with irritable bowel syndrome should take special care to consume a diet that provides adequate amounts of the B vitamins, particularly folic acid. If this is impossible because of the illness, a supplement should be taken. Foods such as bananas and oranges, which are rich in potassium, should be used to replenish the body's supply of this mineral. If constipation is a problem it may be resolved by increasing the amount of dietary fiber.

KESHAN DISEASE

Keshan disease, a serious illness that affects the heart, often leading to disability or death, takes its name from the city in northeast China where it was first identified. Although it does not occur in the United States it is included here because it is an example of a nutritional disease more common in women than in men, and one that demonstrates an important general principle: that a nutritional deficiency by itself may not always lead to illness, but that it may make a person more susceptible to certain illnesses. In China the disease is most often seen in women of childbearing age. It is probably caused by a virus that attacks the heart muscle, but does this only in women who are deficient in the mineral selenium. Yet because selenium deficiency is prevalent in a wide region in China the disease has affected several million young women. Keshan disease therefore requires three conditions: being a woman (although this is not essential, since some men are afflicted); a severe deficiency of selenium; and infection by the virus.

Recognition of the three necessary conditions for Keshan disease, and the discovery that selenium deficiency is a key link in the chain leading to the disease has permitted the Chinese physicians responsible for controlling the disease to eradicate it almost totally by spraying crops with selenium and supplementing populations at risk.

LACTOSE INTOLERANCE

In most of the world's population, lactose (milk sugar) is efficiently broken down in the gastrointestinal tract only during childhood. Therefore, once adulthood begins, the consumption of large amounts of milk or dairy products can cause abdominal pain, flatulence and diarrhea. For most people this is no great problem since the discomfort appears only after relatively large amounts of dairy foods are consumed. In some people, however, particularly Orientals and blacks, even relatively small amounts of lactose-containing foods can cause discomfort, and such people typically shun dairy products. This can present a serious problem for women belonging to these groups since dairy foods are the primary source of calcium in the human diet and calcium is a key nutrient that all women require. The problem can be solved with calcium-containing plant foods, primarily green leafy vegetables. Any woman who cannot consume dairy products should also take a calcium supplement of 500 milligrams per day.

MALABSORPTION

Malabsorption—the impaired or reduced absorption of nutrients from the gastrointestinal tract—occurs in a number of specific diseases of the tract. All of these diseases are associated with diarrhea—and often diarrhea in which large amounts of fat are excreted. Some are more common in women; most are not. However, all are potentially much more dangerous in women than in men because of the nutrients that are lost. Three nutrients that are frequently poorly absorbed in these conditions are iron, calcium and folic acid, all of which, as we have seen, are in short supply in the average woman's diet. For this reason, supplementation of these nutrients is necessary while the disease process is active. After the disease is brought under control a diet rich in these nutrients should be consumed and continued for several years to replenish depleted reserves. Fortunately, most diseases that result in malabsorption can be controlled medically or surgically. Thus, if you have or think you have a condition causing malabsorption it is essential that you seek specific treatment and pay strict attention to replacing lost nutrients.

MIGRAINE HEADACHES

Occasional and even frequent headaches are common in both sexes. However, the type of headache, known as migraine headache, is much more frequent in women.

A migraine headache is often preceded by a short period of depression, irritability, restlessness and loss of appetite. These symptoms may disappear shortly before the headache appears or may merge with it. Usually the pain of the headache is felt all over the head, although it may sometimes be localized to one side or the other. Usually also the pattern of the pain is the same in a given woman, except that if one-sided, it will often alternate from side to side. The headache can last for several hours or even days, and may occur several times a week or only once in several months. The attack is frequently accompanied by nausea, and vomiting occurs in a large number of affected persons.

Any woman suffering from severe recurrent headaches should be carefully examined by a physician. If migraine is the problem, specific treatment is available. This ordinarily involves the use of drugs, and in some recent cases biofeedback techniques have proven helpful. There are also some reports of success with acupuncture. Often, migraine headaches disappear after the age of fifty.

There is no "nutritional treatment" for migraine headache. No vitamin or mineral therapy has proved of any use, nor has any kind of dietary pattern. The most important nutritional consideration for women with migraine is to prevent deficiencies caused by the loss of appetite and vomiting brought on by the condition. Because of these two symptoms, women who suffer frequent migraine attacks will be prone to vitamin and mineral deficiencies, which will exaggerate the normal risk of effects from this and may introduce the risk of certain deficiencies not usually encountered. For this reason, women who suffer from migraine headaches should take a vitamin and mineral supplement, and especially one that includes calcium. This should be done in addition to the therapy prescribed by a physician. Between attacks, a varied diet, emphasizing those nutrients that are in short supply in the diet, should be eaten. During an attack it is important to try to hold down small amounts of high-nutrient-density foods. Liquids in the form of soups are often good for this purpose, and have the added benefit of replacing lost fluid. Fortified grain products, skim milk and low-fat cheese are other useful high-nutrient-density foods for women afflicted by migraine. However, since what works for some women does not work for others, each woman must seek and find the high-nutrient-density foods that she most easily retains.

POSTPARTUM HEMORRHAGE

During the delivery of a baby, the mother will usually lose some blood. Although this blood loss is ordinarily moderate (from one hundred to two hundred cubic centimeters, or three and a half to seven ounces) it can occasionally be extremely heavy (five hundred cubic centimeters or more). Such heavy bleeding commonly occurs if the uterus fails to contract firmly enough with the birth of the baby or if the placenta fails to separate properly. If the bleeding is very severe, replacement blood will be given. For lesser amounts of bleeding (less than a pint) no specific therapy may be used. Whatever the case, it is important for all mothers to have their hemoglobin checked shortly after delivery, since the mother may sometimes not realize how much blood she has actually lost during the delivery. If anemia is then found, iron supplementation should begin immediately. It is a good idea to take folic acid as well, since the bone marrow will be very active in replacing the lost red blood cells. Diet alone is insufficient for correcting this kind of deficiency; it takes too long, lengthens the recovery period, and could mean a reduced iron content of the mother's milk.

SCOLIOSIS

Scoliosis—a lateral (S-shaped) curvature of the spine—is yet another condition that is far more common in women than in men. It usually begins during childhood and may progress rapidly during adolescence. Once adulthood is reached there is usually no further progression. Usually, no specific treatment is necessary for mild scoliosis. For moderate scoliosis exercises and bracing of the back may be indicated. Severe scoliosis may have to be treated surgically.

Weight control and the intake of adequate amounts of calcium are the two major nutritional considerations in the management of scoliosis. Any weight increase above a person's ideal weight range will cause back strain and pain and, in young girls, may even worsen the spinal curvature. Young girls with severe scoliosis may have to undergo a long period of immobility for correction of the curvature, and this will lead to calcium loss from the bones and can hasten the onset of osteoporosis later in life. Under such circumstances—and in fact for any person with scoliosis—high-calcium foods should be consumed, and during the period of immobility itself a five hundred milligram per day calcium supplement should be consumed.

TOXEMIA OF PREGNANCY

Toxemia of pregnancy is a condition characterized by high blood pressure (hypertension), edema (swelling due to fluid retention) and the leakage of protein into the urine. Up to 5 percent of all pregnant women may suffer from some degree of this condition, which is more common in women who have preexisting high blood pressure. In its most severe form the toxemia may threaten the life of both the mother and the infant. Fortunately, severe toxemia (eclampsia) is very rare and even when it does occur can be controlled with proper treatment. However, any woman suffering from even mild toxemia should be under careful medical supervision. Often bed rest at home will control the situation. Sometimes hospitalization may be necessary.

In the past a major component of the treatment of toxemia was salt restriction and the use of diuretic drugs. Neither is necessary and in fact both may aggravate the condition. A normal salt intake and an increased water intake are encouraged and, with bed rest, will often result in an increased urine output and a loss of the edema. It is very important that a woman suffering from toxemia of pregnancy eat an adequate diet and continue to gain adequate weight. Indeed, some experts feel that undernutrition during pregnancy is a major cause of the condition. Although this is not yet proven, undernutrition and poor weight gain during pregnancy may certainly contribute to the disease by making the symptoms worse.

Thus, physicians today feel that any woman suffering from toxemia of pregnancy should consume a diet adequate to maintain the normal weight gain for this time, with a normal salt content and rich in all the nutrients particularly important during pregnancy. Such an approach, coupled with careful medical supervision, will usually control the illness and result in a healthy mother and infant.

Epilogue:
A Longer and Healthier Life

I hope this book has helped toward an understanding of the special nutritional needs of women. As they prepare for childbirth they must build up the nutrient reserves necessary to carry them through that time of increased demand. During pregnancy and lactation they must nourish another life while keeping their own nutrient reserves from becoming depleted. In their middle and later years they continue to have special nutritional concerns. And as if all of this were not enough, women in American society today have lifestyles that often make meeting these special needs more difficult. Smoking, drinking and the contraceptive pill are among these lifestyle factors. Even more important, however, is the constant emphasis on dieting and weight reduction that is now so prevalent among American women and which limits the amount of food needed to supply those vital nutrients of which a woman's body has the greatest need. Finally, there is illness, which puts an added strain on a woman's nutrient demands—an added burden that must be carefully relieved in order to prevent the further depletion of vital nutrients and the further loss of health.

In all of this there are at least seven key nutrients of critical concern to women: calories; the vitamins folic acid, vitamin B_6 and vitamin B_{12}; and the minerals iron, zinc and calcium. The demand for these nutrients is increased during almost every period of a woman's life. Most especially in contrast to the situation with men is that the amount of calories a woman needs can change drastically depending on her stage of life.

We have also seen the constant need for new blood to replace that lost in menstruation, to increase the body's blood volume during pregnancy and to create a completely new blood supply for the fetus—and with this the need for increased amounts of folic acid, vitamin B_{12}, zinc and iron, the first three because they are crucial to making new blood cells, the last because it is an integral part of hemoglobin, the major component of every red blood cell. Thus during childhood and adolescence, when a woman's blood supply is increasing, during her reproductive years when she loses blood every month, during pregnancy when both she and her fetus are making new blood and during lactation when the blood supply of her infant is rapidly increasing—stages that cover the major portion of a woman's life—her requirement for these two vitamins and two minerals will be increased. That three of these nutrients, iron, zinc and vitamin B_{12}, can all be stored by the body is something of which women should take advantage by keeping their body's reserves as high as they can, and should build up their reserves of these nutrients during those periods in their lives—between pregnancy and lactation—when the demands for them are somewhat lower.

With regard to vitamin B_{12}, women who are not strict vegetarians should have no problem, since this vitamin is so prevalent in all foods of animal origin. As for iron and zinc, getting enough is a constant struggle for most women. We have seen that both of these minerals tend to be found in the same foods and that a deficiency of one is often accompanied by a deficiency of the other. The foods rich in these minerals have been given, and will hopefully provide enough variety to satisfy almost any palate. What you as the reader should do is to think about these two nutrients when you plan your meals. Soon the right choices will become automatic. And remember, in the case of iron the requirement is such that if you consume less than 1,200 calories per day (which is not uncommon in women who are dieting) it will be virtually impossible for you to meet it. Under these circumstances you will have to consume fortified foods or take a supplement.

Because folic acid and vitamin B_6 cannot be stored by the body, your intake of these must go up when your requirement goes up. For both of these vitamins, pregnancy and lactation are critical periods because of their increased demands. Additionally, the use of the contraceptive pill, heavy alcohol consumption and especially a combination of both interferes with the metabolism of these vitamins. In fact, deficiencies of folic acid and vitamin B_6 are so common among American women that supplementation during pregnancy and lactation is often recommended.

Calcium may in some ways be the most important nutrient to women. They must pay attention to getting an adequate supply of it throughout their lives, from conception through old age. For the first thirty years of a woman's life calcium is deposited into her bones, where it is stored and which are the structural supports of her body; for the last forty or more years her body loses calcium. After menopause this loss becomes very rapid and may result in osteoporosis with fractures of the hip or spine. For all of these reasons, you must absorb enough calcium to build your reserves during the storage years. During your later years you must minimize the loss of calcium from your body by consuming and absorbing as much as possible. Essential to this is a diet rich in calcium, and the reduction of phosphorus intake at calcium-containing meals. Again this means thinking about calcium as you plan your meals, and remembering that while dairy products are the richest source of this mineral, other foods are also important. (See Table 1, Chapter 8.) Because meat is the major contributor of phosphorus in the American diet, a high-calcium food should be included in meals that do not contain meat, and carbonated soft drinks—many of which contain phosphorus—should be avoided with calcium-containing foods.

If only those vitamins and minerals needed in greater amounts were the major question in women's nutrition, the solution would simply be to eat more food. Unfortunately, such a solution carries the problem of too many calories—a problem that in reality does affect many women who are overweight and many others who perceive themselves as such. Yet facing this is the question of too few calories, which means less food and reduced quantities of the vitamins and minerals, including the six key vitamins and minerals critical to a woman's health. Thus, the nutritional paradox of womanhood is the need for more vitamins and minerals in smaller quantities of food.

The answer to this paradox lies in the kind of foods a woman chooses. The key to success is choosing foods of high nutrient density—those that are at once rich sources of vitamins and minerals and low in calories. Fat, the most dense source of calories and poorest source of other nutrients, should be taken only in the minimally necessary amount. Refined sugar, while not as calorically dense as fat, is also devoid of any other nutrients and hence should also be consumed in moderation, as should alcohol, another "empty-calorie" food. By limiting foods that are high in fat, refined sugar and alcoholic beverages you will be well on the way to a diet that is of high nutrient density. And when you emphasize those nutrients which your body has in shortest supply you will have very nearly completed your diet. The tables in this book should help you in all of these areas, and after a while you should no longer need them. It really isn't very hard to develop a dietary pattern that will satisfy your nutrient requirements without giving you too many calories and which will at the same time give you the satisfaction and pleasure of enjoying the foods you eat.

If you follow the dietary patterns outlined in this book I cannot guarantee you a longer life with fewer illnesses, but I can assure you that the statistics are such that your risk of developing certain illnesses will be reduced and you will be doing everything known to keep yourself nutritionally in the best possible condition. It really isn't difficult, and it can be fun. Most important, unlike many of the things in our lives, it is entirely within your control.

Index